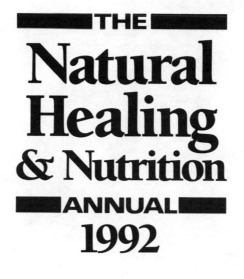

THE
Natural
Healing
& Nutrition
ANNUAL
1992

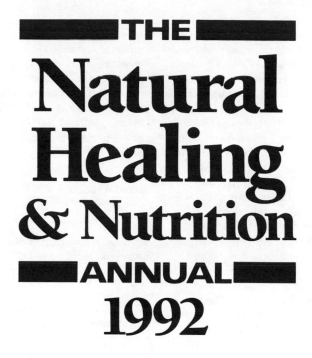

THE
Natural
Healing
& Nutrition
ANNUAL
1992

Edited by Mark Bricklin, Editor,
& Sharon Stocker, Associate Editor,
PREVENTION Magazine

Written by the Staff of Rodale Press

Rodale Press, Emmaus, Pennsylvania

If you have any questions or comments concerning this book, please write:

Rodale Press
Book Reader Service
33 East Minor Street
Emmaus, PA 18098

ISBN 0–87857–980–X hardcover

Distributed in the book trade by St. Martin's Press

2 4 6 8 10 9 7 5 3 1 hardcover

**Contributors to
the *Natural Healing and Nutrition Annual 1992***

Writers: George Blackburn, M.D., Ph.D., Dominick Bosco,
Pam Boyer, Mark Bricklin, Michael Castleman, Stephanie Ebbert, Anne M. Fletcher, Greg Gutfeld, Mor-
ton A. Klein, Steven Lally, Gloria McVeigh, Leslie Ni-
cholson, Charles Norelli, M.D., Cathy Perlmutter,
Paul Perry, Porter Shimer, Adrienne Simons, Maggie
Spilner, Sharon Stocker, Varro Tyler, Ph.D.

Production Editor: Jane Sherman
Cover and Book Designer: Greg Imhoff
Copy Editor: Durrae Johanek
Associate Research Chief, *Prevention* Magazine: Pam Boyer
Office Manager: Roberta Mulliner
Office Personnel: Julie Kehs, Mary Lou Stephen

Contents

■   ■

Nutritional Health Bulletins

Contents

Your Diet and Your Health

Gaining the Upper Hand against Disease

The Frontiers of Medical Care

Everyday Health Concerns

The Science of Positive Living

SUPPLEMENTS AND COMMON SENSE

Some of the reports in this book give accounts of the professional use of nutritional supplements. While food supplements are in general quite safe, some can be harmful if taken in very large amounts. Be especially careful not to take more than these commonsense limits:

Vitamin A	2,000 I.U.
Vitamin B_6	50 mg
Vitamin D	400 I.U.
Selenium	100 mcg

NOTICE

The information and ideas in this book are meant to supplement the care and guidance of your physician, not to replace it. The editor cautions you not to attempt diagnosis or embark upon self-treatment of serious illness without competent professional assistance. An increasing number of physicians are ready to cooperate with clients who want to improve their diet and lifestyle; if you are under professional care or taking medication, we suggest discussing this possibility with your doctor.

Introduction

■   ■

For Good Health, Small Choices Count

Isn't it ironic that achieving our most natural state—good health—seems to take such *unnatural* amounts of willpower? No doubt things were different in more primitive times, when munching on roots and berries, staving off warthogs, and transporting buckets of water from riverside to cave ten times a day kept bodies naturally lean and mean. But in our era, where potato chips, onion dip, and television exist simultaneously, well, good health becomes a thing demanding conscious pursuit.

Luckily, a healthy lifestyle follows a very simple scientific principle: Once the ball is set in motion, it's a lot easier to keep it rolling.

What's more, it doesn't take a mighty shove to get good habits started. In fact, where your health is concerned, the opposite is true: Small choices often count for *more*. Choosing to take a brisk, 15-minute walk, for example, instead of a coffee break five days a week is better for you than an aggressive 2 hours of racquetball once a week. And opting for a piece of fruit instead of the daily afternoon cupcake will get you farther in the long run than consuming an entire head of broccoli at one sitting.

The Natural Healing and Nutrition Annual 1992 is packed with practical information that can help you make better choices where your health is concerned. We take the year's most significant research—targeted from *thousands* of experiments conducted and published each year by leading scientists—and show you how to turn the "big" discoveries into "small" choices that make a big difference in your personal health improvement. We certainly hope you enjoy it—and better health.

The Editors
Prevention Magazine

Nutritional
Health
Bulletins

Nutrients Boost Brain Health

To keep your brain revving at top speed, all you may need is better fuel, a study suggests.

Researchers checked brain function and nutrition status in 28 healthy people over the age of 60. Those with adequate levels of the B vitamin riboflavin had better memory performance, while those with adequate carotene levels were more agile on tests of cognitive (thinking) ability. People with high iron status had brain activity levels (measured by an EEG, an electroencephalogram) similar to young folks in their twenties and thirties—a healthy sign, according to the researchers. Those low on thiamine showed some impairment of brain activity (*American Journal of Clinical Nutrition*).

"It may be that nutrients are as vital for the brain as they are for the rest of the body," says James G. Penland, Ph.D., a research psychologist at the U.S. Department of Agriculture Human Nutrition Research Center at Grand Forks, North Dakota.

You don't need to go overboard in the name of mental gymnastics, though. You can achieve the same nutrient levels as the more successful study participants just by meeting the Recommended Dietary Allowances, says Dr. Penland. A balanced diet that relies on lean meats, fish, fruits, vegetables, and grains can do the trick.

■ High-Fiber Eating Cuts Calories

Sitting down for a healthy crunch of high-fiber cereal in the morning may help you curb the number of calories you take in the rest of the day, a study suggests.

Fourteen volunteers started off their morning with a bowl of one of five cereals—ranging from low to high in fiber content. After 3½ hours, they were guided to a buffet where they were invited to graze on burgers, peanut butter, pickles, corn chips, and other munchies. Those who ate the highest-fiber cereal for breakfast ate about 45 calories less than average at the buffet.

To follow up, the researchers gave another 19 volunteers one of two breakfast cereals—either very low or very high in fiber. As before, people who started their day with the high-fiber cereal ate fewer calories (an average of about 90 fewer) at lunch. Their combined calorie consumption—breakfast plus lunch—was also lower (*American Journal of Clinical Nutrition*).

"Although this was only a short-term study, it suggests that a high-fiber diet like this, continued over the span of a year, could possibly result in a 10-pound weight loss," says researcher Allen S. Levine, Ph.D., of the Veterans Administration Medical Center in Minneapolis. People usually equate eating fiber with feeling full. Surprisingly, though, feeling full was not the reason the fiber eaters ate less. "Even though the people did not perceive they were stuffed, they still consumed less food," says Dr. Levine. This suggests that eating fiber may help you limit total calories without making you feel bloated.

Millions of Women ■
Need More Calcium

Some women who've put menopause behind them may be able to help preserve their bones with extra calcium—something that many researchers didn't think was possible.

That's the suggestion of a preliminary study in which women who were five years or less past menopause saw no change in their rate of bone loss after taking calcium supplements for two years. But some women who were more than five years past menopause did benefit from extra calcium. Their rate of bone loss dropped significantly (*New England Journal of Medicine*). A similar group of women taking a placebo (inactive pill) experienced no effect.

Interesting enough, those women who benefited from extra calcium had been taking in less than 400 milligrams of calcium a day (well below the U.S. Recommended Daily Allowance of 800 milligrams) before the study started. They also were experiencing the most dramatic rate of bone loss. All were given supplements of 500 milligrams per day. (Those women who had a higher initial calcium intake were experiencing less bone loss to begin with and so benefited less from increased calcium.)

"It's a misconception to think that because women within a few years of menopause see no effect from calcium, it wouldn't benefit any menopausal women," says Bess Dawson-Hughes, M.D., chief of the Calcium and Bone Metabolism Laboratory at the U.S. Department of Agriculture Nutrition Center at Tufts University. "It just takes a few years to see the benefits. There are millions of women with low calcium intake who stand to gain from increasing their levels." To bolster your bone, Dr. Dawson-Hughes advises loading up on three servings of calcium-rich foods daily. Translation: Pass the low-fat yogurt, broccoli, skim milk, and low-fat cheese.

■ Potassium Cuts Cholesterol

A banana at breakfast may help give high cholesterol the slip. And a baked potato at dinner may help take the steam out of high blood pressure.

That's the suggestion of a study on the effects of the mineral potassium, which is abundant in these foods.

The researchers discovered this possible potassium bonus when they divided 37 men and women with mild high blood pressure into three groups. One group took 2,340 milligrams of potassium daily (slightly more than the estimated minimum requirement) in supplements. Another group took that plus magnesium, while another took a placebo (inactive pill). After eight weeks, the two potassium groups' blood pressure plunged, compared to the placebo group's. Their cholesterol also took a nose-dive as compared to the placebo group. Those taking both potassium and magnesium, however, didn't do any better than those taking potassium alone (*British Medical Journal*).

"Strong evidence from a number of studies suggests that a diet low in potassium may lead to high blood pressure," says George Webb, Ph.D., associate professor of physiology and biophysics at the University of Vermont College of Medicine. "And some studies have suggested that taking extra potassium may help lower blood pressure. But this is the first study in humans that seems to suggest that getting enough potassium may also help cut cholesterol."

A low-fat diet rich in fruits and vegetables will provide plenty of this essential mineral and is a good idea even if the potassium factor turns out to be less powerful than this study suggests. Top potassium sources include bananas, potatoes, broccoli, tomatoes, and orange juice. Experts say potassium supplements are unnecessary (except in certain medical conditions) because it's so easy to get the mineral in your diet.

Vitamin A Saves Kids' Lives

In form it may look like a plain old pill, but in function vitamin A may be an edible life preserver for kids threatened by deadly malnutrition.

Researchers dispensed vitamin A supplements to more than 15,000 children in an area of southern India where kids are at high risk of vitamin A deficiency and their death rate is high. The amount given (8,333 international units per week) provided the equivalent of the U.S. Recommended Daily Allowance.

In just a year, the death rate among the children receiving vitamin A dropped 54 percent. The research was a collaborative effort of doctors at the National Eye Institute, Bethesda, Maryland, and the Aravind Children's Hospital and the Aravind Eye Hospital, Madurai, India (*New England Journal of Medicine*).

"Poverty, limited food sources, and bad harvests all contribute to the deficiency," says Keith West, Dr.P.H., director of the Vitamin A Program of the Dana Center for Preventive Ophthalmology at Johns Hopkins Hospital. "Supplements are the first line of defense in these malnourished children right now, and they're having a dramatic effect. For the long run, though, improving nutritional education, maternal health, food preparation, and home and community gardening are key in bolstering the diet and elevating A levels."

Treasures from the Sea

Seafood lovers of the world, rejoice!

A plateful of hard-shell crabs can put the pinch on your cholesterol level. And a steaming bowl of clams or mussels may actually help keep your arteries in the swim.

That's the word coming from research at the University of Washington in Seattle.

Once suspected of harboring too much cholesterol, four kinds of ocean dwellers have been put in the clear: clams, mussels, oysters, and crabs.

When a group of 18 men (all with normal cholesterol levels) substituted these seafoods for meat, eggs, and cheese in their diet, their blood fats changed dramatically after three weeks.

One kind of harmful cholesterol (VLDL) dropped by one-third to one-half after a dietary regimen of mollusks (oysters, clams, or mussels). On a crab diet, it dropped by 26 percent. Another kind of harmful cholesterol (LDL) sank 11 to 14 percent when a diet of oysters, clams, or crab was eaten, while a fraction of cholesterol that is highly protective (HDL) actually rose.

But be warned: All these delicacies were served in low-fat recipes, with only vegetable oils added. You can't expect any benefit from fried clams, for instance, when they have ten times the fat content of nonbuttered steamers!

Note this as well: Shrimp and squid flunked out. Overall, the men fared no better on this kind of "surf" than they did on "turf."

Fiber Kicks Kidney Stones

Are you stone-prone? A daily serving of two fiber-rich wheat- or corn-bran muffins or biscuits may be just what the doctor ordered to help your kidneys avoid these painful pellets in the future, research suggests.

When 21 stone-forming patients boosted their low fiber intake of 6 grams per day up to 18 grams using wheat-bran and corn-bran biscuits, they sharply reduced the amount of calcium in their urine. A high urinary calcium level is a major risk factor for stone disease (70 to 80 percent of these stones are made of calcium oxalate).

The patients were already on a special diet high in fluids and low in protein, calcium, and oxalate (because excess calcium and oxalate in the urine are risk factors for stone formation). But the extra fiber seemed to reduce urinary calcium and oxalate even more (*Journal of the Canadian Dietetic Association*).

"We know fiber is healthy for everyone, but according to this study, it seems that increased fiber may be especially beneficial for people at risk for forming calcium kidney stones," says Janey Hughes, clinical dietitian at the Stone Clinic of the Camp Hill Medical Centre, Halifax, Nova Scotia, where the study was done. Experts urge stone-formers to check with their doctors before dramatically increasing their fiber intake.

Caffeine and Exercise Don't Mix

If you're prone to high blood pressure, you might want to make sure you're decaffeinated before you hit the jogging path. Exercise normally causes blood pressure to rise slightly. But a cup of coffee before you start may intensify the surge, according to a study.

Thirty-four men ages 21 to 35 who had normal blood pressure participated in the study. Before straddling exercise bikes, they took either an amount of caffeine equivalent to about 2 to 3 cups of brewed coffee or a placebo (inactive pill). After a period of rest, they rode at various levels of intensity. The experiment was repeated another day with the caffeine takers switching to the placebo, and vice versa.

The caffeine combined with exercise temporarily produced high blood pressure in 44 percent of the subjects tested—more than twice the number who showed this short-term rise in blood pressure from exercise alone. What's more, caffeine caused blood pressure to continue increasing throughout moderate to maximum exercise.

"We were surprised to see the effects of caffeine on blood pressure at all stages of exercise," says William R. Lovallo, Ph.D., associate research career scientist at the Veterans Affairs Medical Center in Oklahoma City. Usually, moderate to heavy exercise dilates blood vessels, boosting blood flow to your muscles and keeping blood pressure from rising too high.

The study was done on men with normal blood pressure, but it's possible the results may hold true for people with high blood pressure, says Dr. Lovallo. "With caffeine increasing blood pressure in moderate to maximum exercise stages, people with hypertension, or at risk for developing it, may want to limit their caffeine on days they plan to exercise."

Men: Beef Up Your Bones

It's not just girl talk anymore. Men, too, should know that calcium is the mineral to mind for building rock-solid bones.

As men age, they too run a greater risk of brittle bones and breakage (though not quite as high a risk as women). But research suggests that taking in about 1,000 milligrams per day of calcium is all it may take for guys to build and keep up their sturdy scaffold. This finding hails from a study of 48 men ages 21 to 79. Researchers found a link between higher calcium intakes and increased bone density at the hip and lower back. This particular link had never been reported before in either men or women (*British Medical Journal*).

That amount of calcium isn't out of reach and is right on par with the U.S. Recommended Daily Allowance— 800 to 1,200 milligrams. You can start boning up at the calcium-rich dairy case. Pick up low-fat and nonfat milk, yogurt, and cheeses. If these foods don't suit you, go green. Dark green veggies, such as kale, collards, and broccoli, all offer ample supplies of calcium. And one of the best things for your bones is—what else?—bones. The soft, edible bones of canned sardines and salmon may also help keep your frame fit.

High C—Healthy Blood Pressure

Raising a glass of orange juice may help lower blood pressure, research hints. Two studies uncovered the same intriguing preliminary evidence—an association between high blood levels of vitamin C (ascorbic acid) and lower blood pressure.

Researchers at the Medical College of Georgia in Augusta looked at the ascorbic acid blood levels of 67 healthy adult men and women (blood levels are a good indication of dietary vitamin C intake). They found that those with the highest levels of ascorbic acid had significantly lower blood pressure than those with the lowest levels. Those with high vitamin C intake had a mean blood pressure reading of 104/65, compared with 111/73 for the others.

In a separate study at the U.S. Department of Agriculture Human Nutrition Research Center on Aging at Tufts University and the New England Medical Center, a similar trend was seen in 241 healthy elderly Chinese Americans. Those with the lowest ascorbic acid levels tended to have the highest blood pressure. Both studies' results were reported at the American Society for Clinical Nutrition's 30th Annual Meeting in Washington, D.C.

The researchers don't know whether a low level of vitamin C in the blood actually causes a rise in blood pressure. Lower vitamin C intake could just be a sign of a less healthful diet overall, which may influence blood pressure. "We can't draw any conclusions yet," says Paul F. Jacques, Sc.D., an epidemiologist at Tufts. "But the association we found certainly deserves further investigation."

There are tons of healthy reasons for including fruits and vegetables in your diet; getting your daily requirement of vitamin C is just one. Good sources include oranges, green peppers, potatoes, broccoli, tomatoes, strawberries, cantaloupe, grapefruit, and spinach.

Diet Beats Breast Cancer Risk

When does a dozen mean more than 12? Researchers from around the world found out when they combined and reanalyzed information on diet and breast cancer gathered from 12 separate studies. Considered as a whole, the studies' data make a stronger-than-ever case for the power of a preventive diet.

The researchers looked at dietary intake of fats, fruits, vegetables, and vitamins in over 10,000 women worldwide. Despite the wide range of dietary patterns and the varying rates of breast cancer around the globe, the study yielded surprisingly consistent findings: a significant relationship between higher intake of saturated fat and higher breast cancer risk for postmenopausal women, and a link between higher dietary vitamin C intake and lower risk for all women (*Journal of the National Cancer Institute*).

The investigators decided to project the healthy benefits of changing women's diets based on their findings. By reducing the proportion of total calories from saturated fat to 9 percent (from current levels of 13 to 15 percent) and increasing fruit and vegetable consumption to give an average vitamin C intake of around 380 milligrams per day, they estimated breast cancer risk could be cut 24 percent for postmenopausal women and 16 percent for premenopausal women. Translated into lives saved: roughly 9,000 per year in the United States.

"These diet changes are certainly achievable," says researcher Geoffrey Howe, Ph.D., director of the epidemiology unit of the National Cancer Institute of Canada. "Simple things like switching from whole to skim milk, reducing intake of butter, eating leaner cuts of meat, and removing the skin from chicken can bring saturated fat intake down to that level."

Vitamin E Reduces Drug Drawback

Vitamin E may offer hope to patients who experience tardive dyskinesia (TD), a powerful side effect of antipsychotic (neuroleptic) medications. TD is an often irreversible condition characterized by involuntary muscle spasms, usually in the face and fingers. In severe cases, it can even involve the respiratory muscles.

At the Baltimore Veterans Administration Medical Center, a small study took place involving eight people with schizophrenia who were on neuroleptic medication. The patients, all with persistent TD, were given either vitamin E or a placebo (inactive pill) with their medication for four weeks.

For the next four weeks the patients switched treatments. The severity of the TD was measured using a scale that gauged involuntary movements. When the patients were taking vitamin E, the scale showed significantly less TD—with five of the eight patients experiencing reductions of 30 percent or more (*American Journal of Psychiatry*).

"This holds implications for anyone on neuroleptic medication, which puts them at high risk for TD," says main investigator Ahmed M. Elkashef, M.D. "In the future, if vitamin E is used much sooner, in a preventive role, we may see much less TD."

Neuroleptic medications have been shown to increase the processing of the neurotransmitter called dopamine in the brain. Increased dopamine metabolism may lead to a greater production of free radicals—highly reactive, unstable molecules that can cause cell damage. The researchers hypothesize that TD may be the result of cell damage in the brain. Vitamin E is an antioxidant: It may neutralize the effects of oxygen-derived free radicals, preventing TD. (*Note:* Patients should not make changes in medication or supplementation without first consulting their doctor.)

Energize Your Afternoon ∎

Here's food for thought: Eating yogurt or a piece of fruit may give your brain a much-needed boost in the late afternoon, a study suggests.

Ten men met four times over four weeks. One day they were given breakfast, lunch, and an afternoon snack (a candy bar). Another day they were given the same— minus the lunch. On a third day they were given break- fast and lunch and a diet soda at snacktime. On the fourth day, they ate the same, minus the lunch. Fifteen minutes after snacktime, the men took tests measuring memory, arithmetic reasoning, reading speed, and atten- tion span. The experiment was then repeated with an- other eight men, with yogurt instead of the candy bar.

In both experiments, when the men had the higher- calorie snack—the yogurt or candy bar—they did signif- icantly better on most tasks. Yogurt was associated with slightly better performance than the candy bar. But sur- prisingly, lunch had little or no effect (*Appetite*). "The snacks seemed especially useful for tasks that required a great deal of attention," says Robin B. Kanarek, Ph.D., a professor of psychology at Tufts University in Massa- chusetts.

Dr. Kanarek thinks yogurt performed marginally better because it is higher in protein (previous studies suggest that protein plays a role in mental performance). But any high-energy snack, such as a piece of fruit, should help, she says.

The snack may help fight the postlunch dip, in which thinking performance sinks to its lowest at 2:00 or 3:00 P.M. Dr. Kanarek doesn't know exactly what happens, but she speculates that hormonal lows in the afternoon may leave us mentally sluggish. "It's much too soon to tell, but a snack may provide the energy needed to stimulate output of these hormones."

∎

The Healthy-Heart Oil

If you've switched to olive oil because you've heard of its cholesterol-busting prowess, you may be getting a healthy bonus. In a comprehensive study, it was also linked to lower blood pressure and reduced blood sugar levels.

The study took place in Italy, a Mediterranean mecca for low risk of coronary disease. Nearly 5,000 Italian men and women ages 20 to 59 were asked what kinds of fats and oils they used in their food and how frequently they used them. The study confirmed that those who used olive oil regularly had significantly lower cholesterol. It also found that their blood pressure was 2.5 percent lower (unlike those who used polyunsaturated fats, who showed no reduction in this heart disease risk factor), and their blood sugar levels were 6.6 percent lower in men (good news for diabetics).

Maurizio Trevisan, M.D., of the school of medicine at State University of New York, Buffalo, finds the results promising. "It looks like we may have found extra benefits from using olive oil in improving the coronary risk profile," he says.

No one really knows how olive oil might do this, but Dr. Trevisan speculates: "Monounsaturated fats [like olive oil] may affect metabolism and production of insulin, which could explain the beneficial effect on both blood pressure and glucose levels."

It's no secret a diet high in saturated fat can drive cholesterol levels up. But in this study, people who frequently used butter (high in saturated fat) had higher levels on all counts—cholesterol, blood pressure, and blood sugar—than those who rarely used it. It may be that using olive oil instead of butter may combat the triple threat. Confirming studies are needed to make that clear, though.

Breast-Feeding Boosts Immunity

Many people already know that breast-feeding offers a new baby an extra blanket of protection against infection, as some of the mother's immune factors are transferred to the baby in the milk. But now research adds an interesting wrinkle: Something in the milk may accelerate the baby's own immune system, giving the infant even more of a fighting chance against sickness.

Researchers at the University of Texas Medical Branch at Galveston have looked at white blood cells found in breast milk. They found that some of these immune cells looked more developed, more mature, than their counterparts in the blood. Recently they discovered that these cells also moved faster than their counterparts in human blood. They believe this activity is due to the presence of a protein in the milk that stimulates the immune system. So it seems likely that this protein, called tumor necrosis factor-alpha, may have important beneficial effects on the baby's immune system.

"It's already widely accepted that human milk is rich in factors that protect directly against infection," says Armond S. Goldman, M.D., one of the researchers. "But we found preliminary evidence that it contains at least one factor that activates the baby's own immune system. We are now examining human milk for similar agents. Once we can narrow it down to a specific agent, we hope to study the actual effects on the recipient of the milk—the baby."

■ In Favor of Fiber

A major reappraisal of fiber's effect on colon cancer risk—drawing from over 37 studies involving more than 10,000 people—adds confirmation that a high-fiber diet may help lower the incidence of that disease. While many of the individual studies showed significant correlations between increased vegetable or fiber intake and lower colon cancer risk, some detected no such correlation.

When researchers analyzed the findings of all the studies, however, they found that diets high in vegetables, fruits, and grains corresponded to a reduction of up to 40 percent in colon cancer risk (*Journal of the National Cancer Institute*).

The varied results of the original studies may have been due to the broad range of methods used and different types of fiber studied. "Instead of focusing on one type of fiber, we looked at a general diet high in fruits, vegetables, and grains," says Bruce Trock, Ph.D., an epidemiologist at the Fox Chase Cancer Center in Philadelphia. "Based on these results, people shouldn't focus on eating just one type. They should take advantage of [many] sources."

Dr. Trock also encourages following the National Cancer Institute's guidelines of eating 20 to 30 grams of fiber per day. One serving of high-fiber cereal, three servings of whole grain bread, four servings of fresh vegetables, and two servings of high-fiber fruit, for example, would provide this amount.

Fiber's positive effect probably doesn't stem solely from replacing fat intake, Dr. Trock says (fat is suspected of raising colon cancer risk). By speeding up passage of the intestines' contents and diluting potential carcinogens, fiber may reduce exposure of cells to cancer-causing agents.

Dr. Trock also advises that people over 50 contact their physician about getting yearly screenings for colon cancer.

B Vitamin vs. Drug Side Effects

Folate, a B vitamin found abundantly in leafy green vegetables, may help reduce side effects of a powerful drug used for rheumatoid arthritis, a study shows.

The drug, methotrexate, is a last resort for people with profound symptoms who haven't responded to other treatments. But it carries side effects severe enough to cause some patients to stop taking it. The researchers decided to try folate because those side effects—nausea, mouth inflammation, abnormal liver function tests, and cell deficiencies in the blood—are similar to the effects of folate deficiency. Also, methotrexate is known to inhibit many of the biochemical processes that require folate.

In a 24-week study, 32 people with rheumatoid arthritis were given, along with methotrexate, either a daily 1-milligram folate supplement or a placebo (inactive pill). In the placebo group, 67 percent experienced some toxicity; 4 experienced symptoms bad enough to stop taking the drug. In the folate group, only 33 percent experienced toxicity, with no dropouts (*Arthritis and Rheumatism*).

"The [folate] seemed to lessen many of the toxic effects—especially gastrointestinal side effects," says Sarah L. Morgan, M.D., a registered dietitian and assistant professor in the Department of Nutrition Sciences, University of Alabama at Birmingham. Although the results are preliminary, the implications are positive.

"Methotrexate is one of the best medications we have for rheumatoid arthritis," says Dr. Morgan. "If we can make it even better by lessening its toxicity, it may become available to more people."

The study participants received prescription dosages of folate, and Dr. Morgan stresses that it should not be used without a doctor's supervision. Furthermore, she says, it's important to maintain close contact with your doctor if you are on arthritis drugs.

A Diet to Bypass Heart Disease

It's right there in black and white. For the first time, angiographic (x-ray) evidence shows how lean your diet must be to prevent the formation of new deposits of cholesterol-laden plaque along artery walls. What's more, the dietary changes needed to have this effect are relatively easy.

Researchers studied 162 men who had recently undergone coronary-bypass surgery; they were chosen because it is known that they're at very high risk of plaque formation. Indeed, it's common for the bypasses to become clogged even after five years or so in these patients.

The men were asked to follow a diet that got 26 percent of its calories from fat. Angiograms of all the men's arteries were taken both at the beginning and end of the two-year study.

Not all the men succeeded in their diets. But those who ate the leanest—less than 23 percent fat—had a negligible risk of developing new occlusions. In fact, 19 out of 20 had no new artery-clogging plaque at all (*Journal of the American Medical Association*).

"It's clear that diet can affect the formation of new coronary lesions," says David H. Blankenhorn, M.D., director of the Atherosclerosis Research Institute and professor of medicine at the University of Southern California. "And the diet choices made by the healthier subjects in the study were not at all tough to do." They simply substituted low-fat meats and dairy products for high-fat versions, while eating more complex carbohydrates, mostly in the form of vegetables, according to Dr. Blankenhorn. The increased protein and carbohydrate calories compensated for the reduced intake of fat. The men still ate heartily, and they didn't lose weight.

Don't Skip Breakfast ■

Munching on a bowl of cereal each morning may help you keep the lid on your blood cholesterol level, a study suggests. A high cholesterol level is a major risk factor for heart disease.

Researchers studied a government survey of the diets of almost 12,000 people. They divided the people into three groups: those who ate any ready-to-eat cereal at their morning meal, those who did not have cereal, and those who skipped breakfast altogether. They found that the cereal eaters had the lowest cholesterol, while the breakfast skippers had the highest. Cereal eaters' cholesterol levels averaged 6.6 points lower than breakfast skippers'.

"We've known that one of the worst things you can do for proper nutrient intake is skip breakfast. But now we have evidence that people who eat a breakfast including cereal have lower cholesterol," says the study's author, John L. Stanton, Ph.D., of Saint Joseph's University in Philadelphia.

Dr. Stanton speculates that it isn't what's in the cereal that lowers cholesterol, but the fact that breakfast skippers may compensate for calories missed in the morning by munching on fatty foods. This may account for their higher cholesterol levels. "Later in the day, they probably weren't making the best food choices," he says. But a cereal eater may feel full and avoid snacking or eating lots of fatty foods later.

Based on these results, Dr. Stanton has some recommendations. "Eat breakfast," he says. Although the morning meal may not be the only factor contributing to lower cholesterol, it was the skippers who fared worst in that department. "And if you already eat breakfast," he adds, "then include cereals." To maximize the health bonus at breakfast, choose cereals (and other foods) that are low in fat and sugar.

Your Diet
and
Your Health

The "Cholesterol 300 + " Attack Plan

You have some routine blood tests done. Days later, your doctor gives you a call to report that everything's just fine—except your blood cholesterol. The level is 330 milligrams per deciliter (mg/dl) of blood, which far exceeds the upper limit of 200 mg/dl recommended by the National Cholesterol Education Program and the American Heart Association. Your risk of heart disease may have just hit the stratosphere.

So what's to be done?

"The knee-jerk reaction of most doctors in this country would be to put you on cholesterol-lowering drugs," says William P. Castelli, M.D., director of the ongoing Framingham Heart Study in Massachusetts. "There's no question that special steps are in order for people with cholesterol above 300 mg/dl. But before you spend money on medication, I say you should talk to your doctor about investing a good six months in a solid cholesterol-lowering diet and exercise program."

Other experts agree. They say that people with sky-high blood cholesterol can make lifestyle changes that, in some cases, can preclude the need for cholesterol-lowering drugs. People who already have heart disease—that is, they've had a heart attack, a blockage documented by an angiogram, a bypass operation, or an angioplasty, or they're on drugs for angina—might not be able to wait six months. They may need to turn to cholesterol-lowering medications sooner. But most others are good candidates for the nondrug plan presented here.

It's worth serious consideration because experts say that any cholesterol reading above 240 mg/dl may place you at high risk of having coronary heart disease. (A 240-plus cholesterol reading by itself does not definitely put you at high risk, but it is a warning sign. As we'll see shortly, other factors play a role, too.) Coronary heart disease is the condition in which major blood vessels leading to the heart are narrowed with cholesterol-containing blockages, called plaque. If a blood vessel becomes completely plugged up, the result is a heart attack.

Occasionally, people with cholesterol levels above 300 mg/dl get them up there by sheer gluttony—in Dr. Castelli's words, "by pigging out on foods like steaks for breakfast, lunch, and supper."

But that's not the typical case. Usually high blood cholesterol is the result of a genetic disorder called familial hypercholesterolemia. The higher your cholesterol is, the more likely it is that the problem is of genetic origin.

"Whether your cholesterol is high because of the way you eat or because you have the worst genes in the world," Dr. Castelli says, "you'll have to follow a diet low in total fat, saturated fat, and cholesterol and get more exercise—whether or not you go on medication. Some people who try the nondrug approach first will be cured by diet alone; others won't be, but they will be better prepared to go on cholesterol-lowering drugs." By being "better prepared" he means you'll need a lower dose of medication, and that decreases the potential side effects of the drug, as well as saving money.

So if you're a candidate for the nondrug strategy, with your doctor's guidance you can give this Cholesterol Attack Plan a try for six months. (Don't attempt this program without letting your doctor know, and be sure to continue with any medications you're currently taking.) It's a multiphased assault on the problem. The more pieces of the package you take on, the more likely you are to chop down your cholesterol reading, possibly with little or no medication. "A successful cholesterol-lowering program consists of making a lot of little decisions all day long," Dr. Castelli says. "It's like saving all of your pennies in a bank account."

Step 1: Verify the Problem

22

■

Make sure your initial sky-high cholesterol reading is correct. Ask your physician to order a repeat blood test (hypodermically drawn) from a reputable laboratory—one that's certified by the Centers for Disease Control for testing blood lipids. You don't need to fast before tests for total blood cholesterol. (Beware of finger-stick tests done with portable cholesterol analyzers. The results are not very precise, although such tests are sometimes used in initial screenings as adjuncts to further testing.)

If the second measurement—which should be made one to eight weeks after the first—is within 30 points of the first, then take the average of the two tests as your cholesterol level. But if the discrepancy is greater than 30 points, a third test should be done within one to eight weeks, and the average of the three tests should be used as your cholesterol level.

If you still come out in the risky zone (240 mg/dl or higher), you should have further testing, called lipoprotein analysis. For this test, you shouldn't have anything to eat for 10 to 12 hours beforehand. Lipoprotein analysis reveals how much of your total cholesterol is the "good" kind (HDL), how much is the "bad" kind (LDL), and how high your triglycerides are. (If a family member has had a heart attack or stroke before age 40, you should have your blood checked for high LDLs or triglycerides, even if your total cholesterol is under 240.)

If your LDL cholesterol turns out to be 160 mg/dl or higher, or your triglycerides are 150 mg/dl or higher, or both, then you're at high risk for heart disease. The LDL cutoff is even lower—130 mg/dl—for someone who already has heart disease or who has two other risk factors. Risk factors include cigarette smoking, high blood pressure, being male (since before middle age, men are much more likely than women to have heart disease), diabetes, HDL cholesterol below 35 mg/dl, or family history of premature heart disease (that is, a heart attack or sudden death before age 55 in a parent or sibling).

On the other hand, it's possible—but very unlikely—that a high total cholesterol reading (even one as high as 300 mg/dl) is the result of having high levels of "good" HDL and safe levels of "bad" LDL and triglycerides. According to Dr. Castelli, there are certain people with HDLs of 80 to 100 who—despite high total cholesterol

23
■

levels—are protected against heart disease. (Have a repeat HDL test if it comes out this high, to make sure it's not a fluke.) If the ratio of total cholesterol to HDL cholesterol is less than 3.5, he thinks there's little worry about heart disease and that you need only to avoid very fatty foods. In most cases, however, having high blood cholesterol is the result of having high levels of LDL.

Be aware, too, that certain diseases—of the thyroid gland, liver, or kidney, for instance—can raise blood cholesterol, as can some medications, such as certain diuretics. Your physician needs to make sure your cholesterol is not related to one of these before starting you on an aggressive diet or medication.

Step 2: Make Some Positive Changes

It's confirmed: You've had all the right tests, and your cholesterol level is still above 300 mg/dl with an LDL level well over 160 mg/dl. Next, devote two months to three smart moves known to cut cholesterol down to size.

Attack the Fat ▶ The single most effective step you can take to lower your blood cholesterol is to cut the amount of saturated fat you consume to less than 7 percent of your calorie intake, down from the American average of 13 percent.

One way is to drop your total fat intake to 20 percent of total calories, which automatically cuts your saturated fat intake way down. People whose cholesterol is high because they've been eating tons of saturated fat may respond to the guideline for the general public to lower fat to 30 percent of calorie intake. But most people with cholesterol above 300 need to cut fat further. Here's how to shoot for the 20 percent mark.

■ Have no more than one serving of lean meat, fish, or poultry a day, limiting portion size to 3 or 4 ounces (the size of a deck of cards).

■ Limit red meat to two or three servings a week.

24
■

■ Have two servings of whole grains, breads, or starches (like pasta and potatoes) with every meal— more if you can afford the calories.

■ Have one vegetarian meal each day. (Combine pasta, rice, barley, and starchy vegetables, such as potatoes, corn, and winter squash.)

■ Each day, substitute two servings of nonfat milk products (such as skim milk and nonfat yogurt) for two servings of fattier ones.

■ Each day, use no more than 2 to 4 teaspoons of added fat or oil in cooking or on foods. (When you do, stick with olive oil, canola oil, or liquid plant oil, such as corn, sunflower, or safflower.) Choose margarine with a liquid vegetable oil listed as the first ingredient. Don't use butter, shortening, or lard.

■ Use only low-fat condiments or toppings—like fat-free butter substitutes, nonfat salad dressings, prepared mustard, horseradish, catsup, chili sauce, relish, and salsa.

Note: Dropping your saturated fat intake automatically lowers cholesterol intake, since the two tend to go hand-in-hand in foods. But to stick with the recommended allowance of no more than 200 milligrams of cholesterol from foods per day, you should also limit egg yolks (which are rich in cholesterol) to no more than one a week. Cholesterol-free egg substitutes or two egg whites can be substituted for one whole egg in recipes.

You should also avoid organ meats like liver because of their high cholesterol content.

Boost Your Fiber Intake ▶ Include between 20 and 35 grams of dietary fiber in your diet each day, using as much soluble fiber as possible. James W. Anderson, M.D., of the University of Kentucky College of Medicine, and others have repeatedly demonstrated that eating high amounts of soluble fiber from sources like oat bran, legumes, and psyllium can help lower blood cholesterol. You just have to remember to increase your fiber intake gradually and drink plenty of water.

■ Eat a bowl of high-fiber cereal daily, preferably one with oat bran or psyllium. (Some research suggests that rice bran may have similar cholesterol-lowering effects.)

■ Slowly work up to having ½ to 1 cup of legumes a day, such as kidney beans, chick-peas, lima beans, lentils, navy beans, or pinto beans. A cup of most types provides about 10 grams of fiber. (You can combine legumes with small amounts of meat, chicken, or fish, mix them with low-fat cheese, rice, or pasta, or add them to hearty salads, soups, casseroles, stir-fries with vegetables, or pita-bread sandwiches with sprouts and low-fat cottage cheese.)

■ Add oat bran to foods whenever you can. One-third cup of oat bran provides about 4 grams of fiber. (Dr. Anderson suggests using oat bran in low-fat muffin recipes, as a meat loaf extender, in soups and stews as a thickener, as an ingredient in blender shakes, baked into breads and rolls, in place of bread crumbs, in pancake batter, and in casseroles.)

■ Consider taking a multivitamin/mineral supplement containing iron and zinc, since high amounts of fiber can interfere with the absorption of these and other nutrients.

Get Aerobic ▶ Work up to two miles of brisk walking a day. Not only can regular aerobic exercise like walking help lower total cholesterol, LDL cholesterol, and blood pressure, it's also one of the few things you can do to raise your HDL cholesterol. Walking is probably the safest aerobic exercise you can participate in.

Exercise can help you lose weight, as well, which in and of itself can help lower total and LDL cholesterol. (Be aware, however, that even skinny people can have high blood cholesterol.)

Step 3: Recheck

After two months of following step 2, have your total cholesterol, LDL, triglycerides, and HDL levels rechecked. If your LDL cholesterol is below 160 mg/dl (or 130 mg/dl if you have coronary heart disease or at least two other risk factors), your triglycerides are below 150 mg/dl, and your ratio of total cholesterol to HDL is under 4.5, then you've found a diet and exercise solution to your problem. Your risk is now normal. Dr. Castelli maintains that as long as your LDLs and triglycerides are this low, and you have enough HDLs, it's okay if your total cholesterol doesn't come all the way down to 200 mg/dl. Keep up the good work. But remember, the lifestyle changes have to be forever or your cholesterol is going to soar again.

"One way to stay on the straight and narrow," says Dr. Castelli, "is to have your blood tested for total cholesterol, LDLs, triglycerides, and HDLs regularly for the rest of your life. I recommend testing every three to four months for the first three to four years, then every six months thereafter."

If your LDL cholesterol still isn't below 160, move on to step 4.

Step 4: Try Psyllium

One way to try to nudge your LDL cholesterol down further is to give your soluble fiber intake another boost—by adding an over-the-counter psyllium supplement to your step 2 diet.

Dr. Castelli's advice is to take a tablespoon of psyllium each day for a month, then have your blood fats checked. (A tablespoon of sugar-free psyllium adds about 10 grams of dietary fiber to your diet.) If the level is still not low enough, take 2 tablespoons a day for a month and have your blood fats checked. (The slow increase allows you to adapt to psyllium's laxative effects. Drink plenty of water. Do not exceed two tablespoons.)

Note: Some people are allergic to psyllium. Stop taking it if you get allergic symptoms: wheezing, itching, or shortness of breath.

If your LDL, triglycerides, and total cholesterol-to-HDL ratio are where they should be, then you have found the program that works for you. Keep it up and have regular blood tests. If your LDL cholesterol and triglycerides are still not low enough—and you really want to do everything in your power to lower blood fats without medication—go on to step 5.

Step 5: Go Vegetarian

For two months, go on a strict vegetarian diet with about 10 percent fat calories, such as the heart disease-reversal diet of Dean Ornish, M.D., described in his book *Dr. Dean Ornish's Program for Reversing Heart Disease*. His research suggests that such a diet, coupled with exercise and stress-reduction techniques (plus quitting, if you smoke), may significantly reverse coronary blockages in just one year. And other research shows that this kind of very-low-fat diet is associated with very low LDLs, triglycerides, and total cholesterol.

HOW TO MAKE THE BIG CHANGES

No one is saying that it's easy to dramatically alter your lifestyle to change your blood fats. But plenty of people have done it—and lowered their cholesterol 100 points. To successfully make such big changes and stick with them, the experts consulted by *Prevention* say:

• Set measurable goals for yourself. Like getting a certain amount of exercise or a set amount of fiber each day. People who do this feel good about their accomplishments, so they want to do more.

• Don't dwell on the negative. Instead of focusing on what you can't have, think about all the things you can have. For instance, instead of lamenting the fact that you can't eat bacon and eggs, think about having whole wheat pancakes or french toast (made with egg whites in a nonstick pan),

Although it's tough to follow a diet like this, Dr. Ornish thinks it's important that people know it's a possible alternative to drug therapy for high blood cholesterol. If you want to consider it seriously, it's important that you check with your doctor first.

In this diet, you continue with all the changes of step 2 but limit fat more, increase carbohydrates, and maintain your level of fiber.

■ Delete all meat, poultry, and fish. Let every meal feature foods containing grains and grain products (preferably whole grains), such as bread, cereal, rice, pasta, and tortillas; fresh or dried fruits; vegetables and greens; beans; sprouts; and egg whites. Tofu and tempeh, which are naturally high in fat, are permitted in moderation.

■ Limit milk products to 1 cup of skim milk or nonfat yogurt a day. Eat no cheese.

---

topped with jam, powdered sugar, or maple syrup . . . or a bagel topped with low-fat cottage cheese and herbs, yogurt cheese, or jelly.

● Think about how much more you get to eat on a low-fat, high-carbohydrate diet. Food intake isn't limited on such diets, so many people say that the menus rarely leave them hungry.

● Do it because you'll feel good, not out of fear. Dean Ornish, M.D., who has developed an effective lifestyle program for reversing heart disease, says that fear—like worrying that you'll have a heart attack—motivates you only for a short time. He emphasizes that people who make the changes find that they stay motivated because they feel so much better.

■ Use no oil or egg yolks and only a moderate amount of sugar and salt. Eat no butter, margarine, shortening, or lard.

■ Limit "taste enhancers" to seasonings like herbs, mustard, or salsa.

■ Take a multivitamin/mineral supplement to ensure you're not missing any nutrients because of the dietary restrictions.

Step 6: Check Your LDL Again

Is it still too high? Don't feel bad. The truth is that many people with familial hypercholesterolemia do wind up needing medication. But at least now you know you've done everything possible to avoid reliance on drugs. And it's possible that after six months of trying, you may need far less medication than you would have otherwise.

"Once you're on cholesterol-lowering drugs," says Dr. Castelli, "it's forever. Therefore, since all of the drugs have side effects, we want you to be on the smallest amount of drug that will be effective." That's why it's still important to stick closely to the Cholesterol Attack Plan while you're on medication.

If your LDLs and triglycerides are now down where they should be, congratulations. (You can now try to reduce the amount of psyllium you're taking.) Your reward for all your lifestyle changes is a healthier heart and longer life.

2   Pour Yourself a Glass of Cancer Protection

One of the lowliest, unlikeliest anticancer factors ever may not be percolating in a laboratory somewhere—it may be sitting in a carton in your refrigerator. It's little old milk. That's the suspicion of researchers from one of the nation's leading cancer centers.

The scientists, of Roswell Park Cancer Institute in Buffalo, New York, conducted a massive study of 3,334 cancer patients and 1,300 comparable subjects without cancer. They asked all the subjects a crucial question: How many glasses of whole milk, 2 percent–fat milk and skim milk did they usually drink each day? Then the researchers looked for connections between the milk consumption and cancer—or the absence of cancer. They also took into account other variables, such as medical history, smoking, alcohol use, and general diet. And their analysis of the data revealed that the milk factor was indeed potent: It was associated with reduced risk of cancer in two intriguing ways.

The Way of All Fat

The first telling connection was that people who drank 2 percent milk had a significantly lower risk of cancer than those who drank whole milk. This was true for five different types of cancer—oral, stomach, rectal, lung, and cervical. A similar pattern of reduced risk was found for those who drank skim milk.

In light of other research, these findings make sense, the scientists say. Several studies have linked fat in the diet to risk of cancer, including cancer of the breast, colon, rectum, and cervix. So in this study it's little wonder that cancer risk rose and fell as the consumption of milk fat rose and fell. (Whole milk has four times as much fat as skim milk; 2 percent has two times as much fat as skim.)

Now, the researchers aren't claiming that any protective effect seen here is due to low-fat milk alone. They suspect that other low-fat food choices play a role, too, since people who drink low-fat milk will probably also prefer other low-fat fare. But there's good reason, the researchers say, to think that milk fat may be a major number in the cancer/fat equation. Whole milk is the third largest source of fat in the average American diet, after ground beef (hamburgers, cheeseburgers, meat loaf)

31

and hot dogs/lunch meats (so says the highly respected study known as the National Health and Nutrition Examination Survey II). And as a source of saturated fat (the type of fat associated with a variety of health risks), milk takes a close second place to ground beef.

The Unknown Force

The second link between reduced cancer risk and milk was even more intriguing than the first. The researchers found that the cancer risk for people who drink low-fat milk was not only lower than that of those who drink whole milk but also was even lower than that of people drinking no milk at all.

This suggests that milk fat may not be the only factor

HOW TO SWITCH FROM WHOLE MILK TO SKIM—PAINLESSLY

Switching from whole milk to skim milk overnight might be more than most people's taste buds can stand. Like a low-salt diet, a low-fat diet sometimes takes a little getting used to. Here are some ways to train your taste buds to love leaner milk.

Try the "step down from whole" approach. Whole milk gets over 50 percent of its calories from fat. The next step down on the fat ladder is 2 percent milk (which is 2 percent fat by weight, but actually gets about 35 percent of its calories from fat).

To start, mix a carton of whole milk with a carton of 2 percent milk. Drink the mixture in place of whole milk for several weeks, until you become accustomed to the taste. Actually, you might surprise yourself and barely notice a difference, especially if you buy low-fat milk with milk solids added.

After a while, you can reduce the amount of whole milk you add until you become accustomed to 2

at work here. If cancer risks were linked to milk fat alone, you'd expect the risk for "milk abstainers" to be lower than that for those who drink low-fat milk.

One possible explanation, say the researchers, is that the nutrients in milk may offer some cancer-protective effect. Other research seems to suggest as much. Calcium, riboflavin, and vitamins A and C are found in milk, and all four nutrients have been linked to reduced risks for several cancers. "Food products are made up of 1,001 biochemical entities," says the study's chief investigator, Curtis J. Mettlin, Ph.D., chief of epidemiologic research at Roswell Park. "And we really don't know what roles many of these play. So it's entirely possible that the key component of low-fat milk is something we haven't even identified yet."

percent milk. Then you can gradually start adding skim milk to your 2 percent milk. Maybe one part skim milk to three parts 2 percent to start—gradually working your way down to pure skim milk, which gets only a little under 5 percent of its calories from fat. That's well under the 30-percent-calories-from-fat guideline endorsed by a number of health organizations, including the National Cancer Institute and the American Heart Association. The process might take several months, but it can probably lead to a permanent conversion.

Go from skim-plus to skim. Add either dry non-fat skim-milk powder or canned evaporated skim milk to regular skim. Concoct a mixture that tastes close to whole milk, then slowly reduce the amount of these additives over a period of weeks. Soon you'll be drinking pure skim—and probably not even notice the difference.

33

Both whole milk and the low-fat varieties contain about the same amounts of these nutrients, so how is it that they're associated with different cancer risks? Perhaps, say the researchers, their beneficial effects may not seem as strong in people who drink whole milk because of the nonbeneficial effects of higher fat intake. Remove some of the fat, and the beneficial effects of the vitamins and minerals may become more apparent.

Reading between the Lines

So can low-fat milk stop cancer cold? No scientist is ready to say that yet. Even this study can only point to statistical associations without establishing proof that low-fat milk does deter cancer. But the study does draw attention to an overlooked cancer-preventing strategy: If reducing dietary fat cuts cancer risk, and if milk fat is a big part of our total fat intake, then decreasing our consumption of whole milk is a smart move. And the study's hint that there may be some cancer-impeding element in low-fat milk makes this strategy seem all the wiser.

These findings are awfully convenient, since major health organizations have been saying for years that trimming dietary fat can head off a lot of other woes, including heart disease and obesity.

So the prudent tactic to employ is to reduce fat in all areas of your diet. And it can all begin with a glass of low-fat milk.

3   Make Friends with Fiber

By George L. Blackburn, M.D., Ph.D.

With all the confusion about fiber, are we losing sight of the most important fiber factor of all?

A lot of people are concerned about whether they're getting the right amount of the two types of fiber—soluble (as in oat bran, legumes, and psyllium) and insoluble (as in wheat bran). They know that one or the other may help protect against high cholesterol, constipation, hemorrhoids, certain intestinal diseases, diabetes, varicose veins, obesity, and colon cancer. So paying attention to the type of fiber does make sense.

But I think that the emphasis on fiber type has swayed us from the most important fiber issue of all: We need to consume more fiber, period. Health authorities agree that this should be our top priority for fiber-conscious eating.

The Big Challenge

The problem is that getting enough total fiber can be really tough. The average American is consuming far less than the National Cancer Institute (NCI) recommendation of 20 to 35 grams of total dietary fiber per day. American women get about 11 grams of fiber a day on average; men average around 18 grams. The strange thing is, low fiber intake is not just a problem for people who don't try very much to get enough—it also can be difficult for those individuals who are conscientious fiber eaters.

As a health-conscious reader striving to follow a low-fat, high-complex–carbohydrate diet, you're probably eating more fiber than the average soul, with a good mix of soluble and insoluble fiber.

But even if you follow the National Research Council's advice to eat at least six daily servings of a combination of grain products—plus five or more servings of fruits and vegetables—you may be falling short on your daily fiber needs.

Let's look at the amount of fiber in a representative day's menu that would more than meet the NCI's serving guidelines.

Breakfast

1 cup cornflakes	0.5 g
½ small banana	1.1 g
¾ cup low-fat milk	0
½ cup orange juice	0.1 g

Snack

1 English muffin	1.6 g
2 pats margarine	0

Lunch

3 ounces turkey breast	0
2 slices whole wheat bread	3 g
1 large carrot	2.3 g
1 small apple with skin	2.8 g

Dinner

3 ounces broiled salmon	0
1 cup green beans	4 g
½ cup spinach noodles	1.1 g
1½ cups iceberg lettuce	0.8 g
1 cup low-fat milk	0

Snack

5 wheat saltines	0.5 g
1 cup cubed cantaloupe	1.1 g

The total fiber for the day, despite meeting the NCI's serving guidelines, is only 18.9 grams. Obviously, even a well-balanced diet can leave you 5 to 10 grams short. So what's the solution?

Fortification Tactics

I recommend the use of "fiber supplements." Not pills, but higher-fiber foods that you can add to your diet as fiber "boosters." Specifically, I advocate that each day people add a 5-gram fiber booster to their regular eating. (And, of course, in this "regular" eating, fiber intake should already be high, especially at the morning meal.) I base that on a recent study showing that people can comfortably, easily, and willingly add an extra 5 grams of fiber to their daily diet.

Take a look at " 'Supplements' to Boost Your Fiber Intake" on page 38. There you'll find a list of 4- to 5-gram "doses" of some of the highest-fiber foods. The idea is to add any one of these highly concentrated sources to your diet each day.

One day you can get your fiber dose from cereal, the next day from legumes, and so on. By eating a variety of fiber boosters, you'll be more likely to get a good mix of different types of fiber. (People who are increasing dietary fiber for a specific medical problem, such as high blood cholesterol or constipation, must consult with their physician and a registered dietitian about the best fiber sources.)

But as long as your basic diet includes a good mix of fruits, vegetables, and whole grains, it's fine if you choose the same fiber booster every day—½ cup of 100 percent-bran–type cereal, ⅓ cup of kidney beans, one pear, or anything else you want. Or you could mix psyllium or wheat bran with juice or water and drink it each morning to get your 5-gram dose. Perhaps the easiest way to get your 5-gram booster is with cereals, since there are so many high-fiber choices. If you like variety, keep four or five different types on hand.

People watching their weight may need to account for the extra calories in their fiber booster. If, for example, you added raisin bran cereal with milk to your daily meal plan, you might have to give up something else—say the English muffin in the menu on the opposite page. Or if you're used to something sweet after a meal, try having a pear or some plums in place of your usual dessert. You may find that weight control is easier when you eat more fiber because you feel satisfied on fewer calories.

For those who want to add more than 5 grams of fiber to their diet, I recommend not doing it all at once. Too much fiber too soon when your system isn't used to it would likely cause gassiness, bloating, and in rare cases, even an obstruction. A more reasonable plan is to up your fiber in "baby steps"—slowly, over weeks, adding fiber in 5-gram increments. Perhaps 5 grams for five or six weeks, then if all's well, another 5 grams for another five or six weeks, and so on, not to exceed 35 grams.

Also, since fiber soaks up fluids, be sure to drink plenty of water when you up your fiber intake—at least eight 8-ounce glasses.

Making It a Habit

No matter how you take your 5-gram fiber supplement—you can eat it, drink it, build it into bread, or make it into muffins—if it's not convenient and tasty, you won't do it for long. It's fine if you have the discipline to add an ounce of bran or psyllium to a glass of juice each morning and down it. But you could also sprinkle bran on your regular cereal or mix it with applesauce. If you don't like legumes all by themselves, add them to a salad. Just be sure that you're getting that extra 5 grams of fiber each day. Like brushing and flossing your teeth, adding your 5-gram fiber booster has to become part of your daily routine. It's something that you do forever.

"SUPPLEMENTS" TO BOOST YOUR FIBER INTAKE

To get about 4 to 5 extra grams of dietary fiber each day, include one of the following:

⅓ to ½ cup of bran cereal, hot or cold

1 tablespoon raw corn bran, or 3 tablespoons raw wheat bran, or 4 tablespoons raw rice bran sprinkled in cereal, fruit, or yogurt

1½ rounded teaspoons psyllium or 2 teaspoons soy fiber mixed with beverages

3 dried figs

1 large pear

3 medium plums

2 medium peaches

½ cup cooked legumes (for example, chickpeas, kidney beans, lentils)

Note: Fiber content may vary depending on brand or variety.

The 10 Commandments of Good Health

4

There are so many nutritional factors out there that are said to be bad for us that some people think this is a good excuse to do nothing. Sugar, fat, additives, calories, cholesterol, fast foods—do we have to maintain 18-hour-a-day guard duty against all of them?

Susan Luke, a registered dietitian and nutrition specialist at the outpatient clinic, Sports Medicine–Boston, came up with the top ten no-nos that most deserve our attention. She surveyed a number of nutrition experts and used her own experience in dealing with clients, as well.

Her choices are given in order of importance, and after each one there's a bracing shot of purely positive advice.

1. Thou Shalt Not Eat without a Plan or a Goal

When you get in your car to drive somewhere, you have a destination or a goal in mind. And you pretty much know how you're going to get there. If you didn't, you'd probably be out of gas on some back road right now instead of reading this chapter.

But how many of us have a plan—a "road map"—for eating a healthy diet that will help us perform at our top potential? If you do, you're one of the fortunate few. Too many, though, have excellent intentions without any sort of real plan. No matter how hard we try to navigate through individual meals, our chances of following the right course day after day are poor.

Action for Today ▶ Develop a healthy nutrition plan. Put some clear principles down in writing, and post them in a highly visible spot so you can follow your map.

2. Thou Shalt Not Exceed the Speed Limit

To give another automotive analogy, if you were traveling by car from coast to coast, you wouldn't plan on making it in one day. Well, it's the same way with your diet. Changing food habits is a 45-mile-per-hour zone. Trying for 90 will only land you in a ditch.

Remember this little jingle: Inch by inch, anything is a cinch.

When you combine that kind of gradual change with the plan we mentioned, you're bound to have a higher chance of success.

Action for Today ▶ Write down a time frame for accomplishing specific parts of your diet plan. Be realistic. In fact, be kind to yourself. If you don't make it easy, you may not make it at all.

3. Thou Shalt Not Go Longer than 5 Hours without Eating

This is an important follow-up to the first two tips. According to Evelyn Tribole, registered dietitian and director of nutrition services at Columbia Pictures Entertainment in Culver City, California, "After 5 hours without eating, you are subject to ravenous hunger and you do not care about health goals and good intentions. It's 'grab what you can,' and you become vulnerable to your eating environment." Tribole feels that people need to eat at planned times so they have a sense of control over their food choices, rather than their hunger having the control.

Wayne Callaway, M.D., a member of the U.S. Department of Agriculture (USDA) 1990 Dietary Guidelines

Advisory Committee, agrees that we need to have regular eating patterns. "There are biological rhythms and hunger patterns that are determined by our eating patterns. If we can get people to eat breakfast, lunch, and dinner in adequate amounts, then appetite patterns will be established and we will eat more regular meals. If one skips meals, the urge to binge is greater."

Action for Today ▶ Keep a food diary and identify your eating patterns. If necessary, revise these patterns so that you consume your food at regular intervals.

4. Thou Shalt Give Fat a Wide Berth

Excess dietary fats are known to cause health problems. The average American is consuming 80 to 100 grams of fat per day. That is equivalent to almost a whole stick of butter every day! In the 1990 Dietary Guidelines, one goal is "Choose a Diet Low in Fat, Saturated Fat, and Cholesterol." The adult diet should include a maximum of only 30 percent of calories from fat. This would be 67 grams of fat for a 2,000-calorie diet.

Keeping that 67 grams of fat in mind, William Castelli, M.D., director of the Framingham Heart Study, suggests that we read labels and begin to count our fat intake. Of those 67 grams of fat, only one-third (22 grams of fat) should be saturated. It is the saturated fat in our diet that plays the most havoc with our health. Saturated fat is found in all animal fats and the tropical fats: coconut, palm, and palm-kernel oils.

Today more and more foods have nutrition labeling. While saturated fat might not yet be on the label, total grams of fat is listed. Getting that number down to the 60- to 70-gram level is a good start. (Eventually working down to 50 to 60 grams of fat a day is ideal.) To do that, you have to become label-savvy. Dr. Castelli says, "Today because of modern food technology, we have the ability to find substitutes that were never available before." We have choices, and if you count grams of fat, you should discover that you can work in your favorites ... in moderation.

Action for Today ▶ Establish a fat budget for yourself based on 50 to 70 grams of fat a day. Begin to look at the fat content of the foods you eat, and actually visualize the amount of fat in a gram. The weight of a standard paper clip is about one gram. So buttering a slice of toast adds about 1 gram. Two to three peanuts adds another. Modify some of those choices to lower-fat variations.

5. Thou Shalt Not Skimp on Produce and Grains

On the one hand we are eating too much fat, and on the other hand we are consuming too few complex carbohydrates. Let's flip this around. The long-standing basic four food groups recommend two servings a day of fruits, two servings of vegetables, and four servings of grains (bread or pasta, for example). The 1990 Dietary Guidelines have increased these numbers to two fruits, three vegetables, and six grains. These products are high in complex carbohydrates, fiber, and many vitamins and minerals.

Unfortunately, food consumption statistics from the USDA Hanes II study show that the average woman age 19 to 50 is consuming only 1 cup of cooked vegetables and one medium serving of fruit per day. Mary Abbott Hess, registered dietitian and president of the American Dietetic Association, states that there is a "trend toward encouraging the use of more fresh fruits, vegetables, and whole grains. In restaurants there is a shift toward a greater proportion of the appetizers and entrées being the complex carbohydrates."

Action for Today ▶ Eat more vegetables, including dry beans and peas, as well as more fruits, breads, cereals, pasta, and rice.

6. Thou Shalt Not Be a Member of the Clean-Plate Club

So many people clean their plate today because of old messages they received as children. Today we need to eat based on our present needs, not on old tape recordings playing in our mind. Tribole feels that this is one of our biggest problems, "especially when eating out. We get twice what we need. If people could learn to modify this issue, they could eat whatever food they want; just eat 50 percent of it."

Action for Today ▶ Examine your need to clean your plate. Instead eat based on healthy eating goals.

7. Thou Shalt Not Try to Be Too Thin

Wanting to look good and be reasonably trim is a sensible goal. But wanting to look like a fashion model isn't. Models are usually very young, diet too strenuously, and still need to have the right genes to achieve that special look—if only for a few years. And that look is neither normal nor healthy for the great majority of women.

John Foreyt, Ph.D., director of the Nutrition Research Clinic at Baylor College of Medicine in Houston, says, "According to a recent survey the average woman is 5 feet, 3½ inches tall, 134 pounds, with a dress size of 10 to 12. She wants to be 5 feet, 4½ inches tall, 123 pounds, and a dress size of 8. She wants to be 11 pounds thinner. On the other hand, the average man is 5 feet, 10 inches tall, 172 pounds, with a 33-inch waist. He wants to be 5 feet, 11 inches tall, 171 pounds, with a 33-inch waist." Dr. Callaway, a leader in the field of obesity research, feels that, "We are victims of a distorted culture, and not just our genes."

Action for Today ▶ Recognize the body shape that you inherited. Accept this shape and feed it a healthy diet to achieve good health.

43
■

8. Thou Shalt Not Try to Lose Weight without an Exercise Program

Most people focus on food when trying to lose or maintain their weight. Diane Morris, Ph.D, a registered dietitian previously at the University of Massachusetts Medical Center, now at the University of Manitoba, Winnipeg, finds that when questioned, most people have given some thought to their food choices for the day, but few have thought out their exercise plan. But University of Massachusetts studies showed that when individuals were divided into four groups, the group that lost the most weight was the group that combined a low fat intake with an exercise program. According to Dr. Morris, "A low-fat diet with exercise helps protect lean body mass, which is metabolically active tissue, and promotes fat loss."

Losing weight and keeping it off is tricky. Research continues to tell us that exercise is an important key to long-term success, but many people find it difficult to work exercise into an already packed schedule. If you are serious about losing weight and keeping it off, then you'll have to reorganize and treat yourself to increased physical activity.

Action for Today ▶ Begin an exercise program of choice. Start slowly. Do just enough today so you look forward to doing it again tomorrow.

9. Thou Shalt Not Skimp on Water

Water has been termed the forgotten nutrient. The daily turnover of fluid in the body exceeds that of any other nutrient. Because it is essential to so many body processes, adequate water must be available in the body at all times. On average a total of 2 to 3 quarts are lost every day. Based on these losses, a minimum of 2 quarts of fluid should be consumed each day. The remaining fluid needs will come from the liquids found in our solid foods.

"Unfortunately, most of our fluid needs are met by

flavored fluids with lots of calories and not many nutrients," states George Blackburn, M.D., Ph.D., chief of the Nutritional Metabolism Laboratory at New England Deaconess Hospital, Boston. "We need to break that habit by consuming a cup of water before we drink the other. The average person is a pint [16 ounces] short on water each day, putting stress on the kidneys."

Action for Today ▶ Make a conscious effort each day to drink 1 quart (4 cups) of water along with 4 cups of a variety of flavored fluids, such as juices and low-fat milk.

10. Thou Shalt Not Give Food Magical Powers of Good or Evil

There is no doubt about it: A carrot is a healthier snack than a piece of candy. But snacks—or even whole meals—are only small components of your overall diet. Within the framework of a daily diet, there is room for almost anything—in small amounts.

The problem with categorizing all foods as either good or bad is that it gives them a kind of power they really don't deserve. If you should eat a bit of food on your personal "bad" list, you may think of yourself as a bad person. A failure at eating well. A person with no willpower.

Don't give food so much power to control your mind.

In the course of a week, there are few people who can't eat a couple of pieces of candy or other indulgences and still have excellent overall diets. Some foods may even surprise you when you check the facts: McDonald's, for instance, has a shake with less than 2 grams of fat. Black-and-white thinking is simply unrealistic. There is, after all, just one shade of white and one shade of black. Then there are thousands of shades of gray. What we need to learn is to eat in the light gray zone.

Action for Today ▶ Recognize that you can eat anything you want. Some foods are healthier than others, and you should eat more of those.

45
■

5 Researchers See Vitamin C as Cancer Foe

In a little auditorium in Bethesda, Maryland, about 130 scientists from all over the world—from Tokyo to Berkeley—held a meeting that was cosponsored by none other than the government's National Cancer Institute (NCI) and National Institute of Diabetes and Digestive and Kidney Diseases. The topic of discussion: the biological effects of vitamin C and their possible connection to cancer.

"Many of us were aware of research suggesting that vitamin C may have an effect on cancer," says Donald Henson, M.D., program director of the early detection branch at the NCI. "We don't want to turn away from anything that may be promising. So we wanted to give researchers an opportunity to share their results, and the National Cancer Institute wanted to learn the state of the art in fundamental research in vitamin C and cancer."

"The conference opened some eyes," says Gladys Block, Ph.D., an NCI epidemiologist (a scientist who studies the health of various groups of populations).

"Several people there said to me that they came into the meeting skeptical and came out very impressed with the studies presented. There's a lot of very solid, impressive research now."

Here's a progress report on what these experts are uncovering about the potential for fighting cancer with C.

Viable Deterrence

For years studies have shown that diets rich in vitamin C are associated with a lower risk of several kinds of cancer. And now an expert review of the evidence has pinpointed where the strongest connections lie.

In research of her own, Dr. Block took a close look at all these studies and presented her findings at the conference. She summarized 46 separate population studies that estimated people's dietary intake of vitamin C and examined how often they got cancer. Of these 46 population studies, she found 33 gave strong evidence that people with diets containing the highest amounts of vitamin C had the lowest risk of cancer.

"The evidence for a protective effect of vitamin C was especially strong in cancer of the mouth, larynx, esophagus, stomach, pancreas, rectum, and uterine cervix," she says. "And there is increasing evidence of a role in preventing lung cancer."

Some of the studies looked specifically at the link between breast cancer and several dietary factors, including vitamin C, fiber, saturated fat, and beta-carotene. As other research has shown, saturated fat was found to increase breast cancer risk. Surprisingly, though, intake of vitamin C was just as strongly linked to breast cancer, but as a protective factor. Women who got the most vitamin C in their diet had the lowest risk of breast cancer. And women who got the least C had the greatest breast cancer risk.

Dr. Block also analyzed 29 other studies reporting on fruit consumption and cancer rates. Of those studies, 21 showed that cancer rates were much lower in people who ate the most fruit (a major source of vitamin C).

Population studies like these, however, aren't conclusive, Dr. Block points out. In many cases, vitamin C and fruit intake were estimated, which is a less certain process than testing blood levels of the vitamin directly. Also, she says, fruits rich in vitamin C often contain other nutrients that may fight cancer, like beta-carotene and folate. So it's tough to tell exactly what is causing the lower cancer rates. But, she adds, "I do think the evidence is strong enough for me to say that for prevention of some cancers, vitamin C probably makes a difference."

Other research presented at the conference also ex-

47

plored vitamin C's prevention potential and came up with intriguing results. Here's a sampling.

The Colon Cancer Connection

Low levels of vitamin C in the diet may increase the risk of getting colon cancer. That, at least, is the implication of a study conducted by Robert A. Jacob, Ph.D., of the U.S. Department of Agriculture Western Human Nutrition Research Center in San Francisco.

Dr. Jacob reports that low vitamin C intake in eight healthy men seemed to increase their level of one kind of fecal mutagens, substances normally found in the colon that are thought to play a role in colon cancer. (In test tubes, fecal mutagens damage normal cells' DNA, believed to be a crucial step in cancer. No one knows for sure just yet whether they have this effect in the body.) At least three other studies have suggested a link between vitamin C and fecal mutagens.

The men were living at the research center, eating a strictly controlled diet. On this diet, their daily vitamin C intake (derived from supplements) was varied over time from a low of 5 milligrams (which is just low enough to cause scurvy) up to 250 milligrams.

At the same time, the group's fecal mutagens were being carefully measured by John H. Peters, Ph.D., using sophisticated techniques in his laboratory at SRI International in Menlo Park, California.

"When some of the men were on 5 milligrams a day, the level of fecal mutagens rose significantly," Dr. Jacob says. "And they fell back down when vitamin C was increased to 60 or 250 milligrams a day. In other subjects, the mutagen levels remained stable regardless of the vitamin C intake. So we don't know for sure what effect vitamin C will have on each individual."

There are so many factors involved in colon cancer, it's still very difficult to say whether vitamin C can short-circuit its development. "But our results clearly show these mutagens are affected by vitamin C intake in some people," says Dr. Jacob. "And that's a good clue in the search for a possible preventive strategy."

Effects on Tumor Growth

Vitamin C may prevent or delay the growth of tumors triggered by excess doses of hormones, at least in animals. Joachim G. Liehr, Ph.D., professor of pharmacology at the University of Texas Medical Branch in Galveston, found that vitamin C inhibited tumor growth in hamsters that had two forms of estrogen implanted under their skin. One was a known carcinogen: DES (diethylstilbestrol), the drug widely prescribed for miscarriages in the 1950s and 1960s, which has since caused cancers in many daughters of women who took it. The other was estradiol, a form of estrogen in humans and animals that is linked to cancer.

When these agents were given to the test animals in cancer-inducing doses, most of them developed tumors. But when vitamin C was given along with the hormones, only about half as many animals got tumors.

"This is a significant difference," says Dr. Liehr. If such a finding holds true in humans, it means that vitamin C might be used to increase the safety of certain hormone-containing drugs or reduce the cancer risk of naturally occurring hormones. Dr. Liehr suspects that vitamin C may protect healthy cells against hormone damage, or block harmful substances generated by the estrogens.

Animal Studies Encouraging

In animals, vitamin C can block skin cancer caused by ultraviolet light. That's the upshot of one of several animal studies by Linus Pauling, Ph.D., and his colleagues at the Linus Pauling Institute of Science and Medicine in Palo Alto, California. Being exposed to too much ultraviolet light (whether from the sun or any other source) can cause skin cancer in both people and animals. But in this study, irradiated hairless mice getting large doses of vitamin C had only one-fifth the incidence of malignant skin tumors as those getting no vitamin C.

In another study by Dr. Pauling, high doses of vitamin C delayed the formation of breast tumors in mice

49

bred to develop breast cancer. Tumors took 125 weeks to appear in the treated mice, compared with 83 weeks in untreated mice.

"The Pauling studies are a good beginning," says Dr. Henson. "His results are extremely encouraging, but they should be confirmed in other laboratories."

B and C: Beneficial Together?

The combination of vitamins C and B may have a unique cancer-fighting effect. That's the news from researchers from the Mercyhurst College Cancer Research Unit in Erie, Pennsylvania, and Roswell Park Memorial Institute in Buffalo, New York. In their experiments, 40 mice were injected with cancer cells. Twenty of those mice were also injected with a special form of vitamin C and vitamin B. Fifty percent of the mice that got the vitamins were still alive and tumor-free after 60 days. All 20 of the other mice died within 19 days.

The head researcher on this study, Eymard Poydock, Ph.D., says that the vitamin C has the ability to break down the vitamin B molecule, releasing cobalt at the core of the B. Cobalt itself has been used in conventional cancer therapy. So she speculates that it's the cobalt that's deterring tumor growth.

"Of course, you can't extrapolate from mice to humans," Dr. Poydock says. "But these results strongly suggest a need for human studies as soon as possible."

Treating with C

"Treatment of cancer with vitamin C is very controversial," says Dr. Block. "Certainly, no one would suggest that vitamin C should be used alone. But there are a number of animal studies—some of which were presented at the conference—that suggest that there may really be some anticancer effect."

Animal studies also suggest that vitamin C, used in conjunction with conventional therapies like radiation, may reduce the toxicity of the therapies. "It's very significant if it's true," says Dr. Block. "A lot of conventional therapies are so toxic to the body that you can't give a high enough dose to really kill the cancer. Vitamin C might make it possible to get effective high doses." For example:

■ Paul Okunieff, M.D., associate professor in the Department of Radiation Medicine at Massachusetts General Hospital, reported at the conference that in his research vitamin C reduced the toxic effects of radiation treatments on the skin and bone marrow of mice. When the animals received vitamin C, they were able to tolerate higher radiation doses, which permitted better tumor control.

■ In metastatic (spreading) skin cancer in mice, Gary G. Meadows, Ph.D., a researcher at the National Cancer Institute's experimental immunology branch, found that vitamin C supplementation inhibited cancer growth and cancer spread, boosted the positive effects of chemotherapy, and increased the survival of the animals.

■ Hiroshi Kan Shimpo, Ph.D., of Fujita Health University in Japan, was interested in the cancer drug doxorubicin. It's been shown to fight a variety of cancers but unfortunately can sometimes be lethal because it does damage to heart muscle in some people. In his research, Dr. Shimpo found that vitamin C reduced doxorubicin toxicity in mice and guinea pigs, and prolonged their life spans.

How C Does It

Scientists are engaged in detective work to unlock this mystery: How might vitamin C affect cancer?

Investigators believe that the guilty parties in many cancers are "free oxygen radicals," destructive oxygen molecules. Free radicals can be formed in the body by anything from normal body processes and infections to cigarette smoke and air pollution. Scientists think that under the right conditions, free radicals can cause cell damage that may trigger the growth of cancer. Vitamin C (like other antioxidants, such as vitamin E, beta-carotene, and certain chemicals), however, can neutralize free radicals, reducing the cell damage. So one theory is that vitamin C neutralizes enough free radicals to avert cancer.

There are other theories as well. The nutrient, for example, may stimulate the immune system and help the body's own natural defenses. Vitamin C is very concentrated in our white blood cells, part of our defense system. It is also needed for the body's production of collagen, a substance in our tissues that may be important in keeping cancer cells from spreading. "What came out of the meeting was that vitamin C has many biological effects, apparently unrelated to its normal role as vitamin," Dr. Henson notes. "We have very little understanding of those effects."

One study that examined vitamin C's antioxidant properties was conducted by Balz Frei, Ph.D., assistant professor of nutrition at the Harvard School of Public Health in Boston. In this work, he actually arranged for vials of fresh human blood plasma to "smoke" cigarettes.

Fresh plasma containing a normal amount of vitamin C was put into a flask, and a vacuum was created to draw in smoke from a lit cigarette. (Cigarette smoke is known to contain large numbers of oxidizing free radicals.) Afterward, the plasma was analyzed for levels of oxidized fats (fats damaged by free radicals and suspected of causing cancer). Dr. Frei found that as long as there was vitamin C in the plasma, no oxidizing of fat took place. But as soon as the vitamin C was used up, the oxygen damage to fats occurred. There is some evidence that the same process could happen in human lungs.

However, this experiment did not address the question of whether the oxidized fats really cause cancer. But if they do, as scientists suspect, "then this study would suggest that vitamin C is a good anticarcinogen," says Dr. Frei.

The Future of C

"It's very important to remember that these human, test-tube, and animal studies are just a beginning," says Dr. Henson. "Right now there's no scientific basis for recommending vitamin C for the treatment of cancer. More research is badly needed." If you're a cancer patient, you should talk to your physician or nutritionist before making any changes in your dietary regimen.

"For cancer prevention, though, the current research suggests very good reasons for ensuring that you're getting adequate amounts of vitamin C in your diet," says Dr. Block.

Several scientists say they suspect the U.S. Recommended Daily Allowance for vitamin C is too low. One of them, Dr. Frei, comments, "I don't think that means megadoses are needed—there's no scientific basis for that. But I think that slightly increasing the USRDA wouldn't hurt. Instead of 60 milligrams a day, 150 to 250 milligrams would maximize body levels. It would also provide enough vitamin C for smokers and pregnant women, who use it up more rapidly." He adds, "I personally get about 150 milligrams of vitamin C a day by drinking extra orange juice. I don't take supplements." Other researchers, however, say that they do take extra C.

What's next? "The NCI plans to invite some of the conference speakers back to present their data on an individual basis," says Dr. Henson. "We would like to stimulate additional research concerning vitamin C's biological actions and its relation to cancer."

"Vitamin C appears to be a simple and cheap intervention," says Dr. Frei. "In terms of benefiting public health, this research may have enormous implications."

6 Knock Out Cholesterol with Niacin

The B vitamin niacin is getting a lot of attention at some prominent heart disease centers these days. That may surprise some people, considering all the hoopla over the new prescription cholesterol-lowering drugs. But it seems that more and more often, when high cholesterol levels require a powerful taming agent, the choice among top cardiologists and other doctors is niacin.

Kicking Cholesterol with Drugs

Most doctors follow a three-step process in deciding when to give you cholesterol-lowering agents. The steps were laid out by the National Cholesterol Education Program (NCEP). The first step is a blood test for your total cholesterol. If your level tops 240 milligrams/deciliter (mg/dl), then your doctor will go to step two—testing your levels of LDL, the "bad" kind of cholesterol. Particles of LDL are the "delivery trucks" that deposit cholesterol in your arteries. If your LDL is over 160 (or 130 if you have coronary disease or other risk factors, such as heart disease in your family), your doctor will recommend you work to bring your LDL down. Doctors don't always treat high cholesterol if a lot of it is HDL cholesterol, the "good" kind that hauls cholesterol out of your bloodstream.

Step three is a low-fat diet (less than 30 percent of calories from fat). It includes lots of fresh fruit and vegetables, less meat, no butter, and more low-fat dairy products. If your LDL resists a low-fat diet for six months, then you're a candidate for drug therapy. That's where niacin, or nicotinic acid, comes in.

A Powerful Track Record

Physicians got their first glimpse of niacin's potential from a second look at an old study—the Coronary Drug

Project, begun in 1966. Among 8,300 men who'd had heart attacks, only subjects who received niacin to lower cholesterol (out of four drugs tested) had fewer nonfatal heart attacks over five years. But the real payoff came 15 years after the start of the study. A recheck revealed 11 percent fewer deaths in the niacin takers, who lived an average 1.6 years longer than their studymates. Since this study, no other cholesterol-lowering agent has been found to help people live longer.

Ever since that finding, researchers tested niacin in patients with heart disease, and it usually got high marks. In one trial, researchers from Case Western Reserve University Medical School in Cleveland gave 1 gram of niacin a day to 55 people with heart disease and borderline high cholesterol. The niacin users raised their cholesterol-fighting HDL by an amazing 31 percent after about seven months. Total cholesterol—not in the dangerously high zone in this study—didn't change in the subjects. And there were no changes in any cholesterol measure in an untreated comparison group.

Another study at Beth Israel Hospital in Boston involved 101 people with heart disease taking varying amounts of niacin for about one year. The average dose was 1½ grams a day, achieving a 13 percent cut in total cholesterol and a 31 percent increase in HDL cholesterol.

Experts' First Choice

Although niacin is just one of the agents doctors can choose from, specialists at major medical centers say there are two reasons why they prefer to prescribe niacin most of the time.

First, niacin performs better than most of the other cholesterol-lowering (actually, LDL-lowering) agents recommended by the NCEP. Niacin goes to work in your liver, where it short-circuits the LDL-production process, cutting back on the "deliveries" of artery-encrusting cholesterol. By comparison, the drugs cholestyramine and colestipol work in your intestines. There they tie up cholesterol by-products, setting up a chain reaction that

55

forces your liver to pull LDL out of your blood. These drugs, called bile-acid binders, are almost as effective as niacin in reducing LDL. But niacin also lowers triglycerides, another harmful blood fat, while bile-acid binders can raise triglycerides.

Lovastatin works on cholesterol factories in your liver, as niacin does, and may produce an even larger slash in cholesterol levels. But whether it has niacin's potential to prevent coronary heart disease—either reducing heart attacks or lengthening life—is unknown because lovastatin has only been on the market since 1987. (Another blood-fat drug sometimes prescribed is gemfibrozil. Gemfibrozil lowers triglycerides but has only a modest effect on HDL and LDL.)

Thomas G. Pickering, M.D., professor of medicine at Cornell Medical Center in New York, is one of the specialists who choose niacin. In the month or two it takes Dr. Pickering's patients to get up to a full dose, niacin brings their cholesterol levels down by 10 to 20 percent. For many, that's enough to position them in the safety zone.

The second niacin benefit mentioned by all the experts is cost. Niacin bought in supermarkets and health-food stores costs as little as $5 a month. Prescription cholesterol-lowering drugs cost between $43 and $154 for a month's supply. Michael Cressman, D.O., director of the lipid clinic at the Cleveland Clinic in Ohio, points out that bringing your cholesterol levels down is just the beginning. Keeping cholesterol down is a lifetime commitment to drug therapy. So a monthly saving that seems modest at first, multiplied by a lifetime of monthly purchases, adds up to a substantial difference in cost.

Not an At-Home Remedy

But keep in mind that in order to have its powerful effect on blood fats, niacin has to be taken at such high doses that it is no longer considered just a vitamin—it's a drug. And like many drugs, niacin not only can bring harmless but annoying side effects, it also may sometimes be toxic, taking a toll on your vital organs. In a small percentage of cases, niacin can cause liver damage, usually temporary abnormalities that can become permanent if not found and treated. Niacin can also push people inclined to blood sugar problems, peptic ulcer, or gout into full-fledged illness.

Doctors who prescribe niacin often do routine tests to head off these complications. Like many doctors, whenever Dr. Pickering tests cholesterol levels in patients on niacin, he does three blood tests: liver function, blood sugar, and uric acid (for gout). The first battery of tests comes after one month on niacin, then every four to six months, depending on how each patient is doing. Abnormal liver tests (advance warning but not actual damage) occur in less than 5 percent of his patients, Dr. Pickering says. If any blood tests are abnormal, he cuts back on the dose of niacin or stops it altogether and prescribes a second or even a third drug. You shouldn't take niacin at all if you have diabetes, gout, peptic ulcer, or liver damage—conditions you may not even know you have until your doctor uncovers them. That's why you should never take niacin on your own. Cholesterol-taming niacin is 100 times stronger than the amount your body normally needs each day. Niacin might not hurt you if you took a very low dose, say, 100 milligrams a day. But at low doses, niacin doesn't do a thing for cholesterol levels.

Bile-acid binders have the least potential for toxicity because they stay in your intestines and pass out of your body. Lovastatin, which can damage your liver because it targets that organ as niacin does, also requires periodic liver tests. Experts are cautious about lovastatin because its potential for causing other serious complications won't be known until it's been in use for another five to ten years.

Wider Use Expected

Although no one has polled family physicians, Frank Sacks, M.D., a cardiologist at Harvard Medical School, believes niacin is not used as widely as it could be. The biggest obstacle? Dr. Sacks believes it's patients' refusal to take niacin because of its side effects—mainly flushing, itchy and tingling skin, rash, and headache. In the Case Western study, 40 percent of the subjects dropped out because of niacin-related discomforts.

NIACIN'S A POTENT TEAM PLAYER

Cardiologists are customizing their cholesterol-lowering treatments by combining niacin with prescription drugs. Several studies in recent years have lent support to the evidence that, in some cases, pairing niacin with a drug creates superior therapy. At a meeting of the American Heart Association, researchers reported a new study in which the B-vitamin/drug partnership not only eased cholesterol traffic in the blood but also reduced cholesterol gridlocks on artery walls.

One study at the University of Washington, Seattle, involved 120 men with classic warning signs of heart disease: high blood levels of blockage-promoting LDL cholesterol, heart disease in the family, and symptoms like chest pain. For 2½ years, some of the men took the cholesterol drug colestipol plus niacin, and some took colestipol with another anticholesterol drug, lovastatin. A third group got conventional treatment. Before-and-after artery pictures showed that blockages shrank in 11 percent of the conventional-treatment group but grew in 46 percent. By comparison, in both combined drug therapy groups, 35 percent of blockages improved and only 23 percent got worse.

Experts emphasize that larger studies, spanning many years, are needed before the long-term effects of niacin combined with its anticholesterol allies are known for sure.

On the other hand, patient boycotts aren't confined to those taking niacin. Up to 60 percent of people who try bile-acid binders complain about gas and constipation, and doctors have trouble getting people to take enough to be effective. Dr. Cressman finds some people just refuse to swallow two or three scoops of the powders each day. (Lovastatin has few side effects.)

But niacin's side effects can be circumvented. Dr. Sacks says this was demonstrated by the Beth Israel Hospital study, in which he was an investigator. After about one year, amazingly few people dropped out of the trial because of niacin's side effects.

Several techniques helped the subjects in this study handle enough niacin to knock down their cholesterol levels. For one thing, they started with low dosages (100 milligrams twice a day) and increased to as much as 1,000 milligrams twice a day over a period of one to two months.

Also, taking aspirin seemed to relieve the side effect people complain about most—skin flushing—although doctors aren't sure why it works. Dr. Pickering advises taking one aspirin ½ hour before each of two daily niacin doses until your body has gotten used to the vitamin and flushing disappears completely. (People who have stomach ulcers or who are taking a blood-thinning drug can't take daily aspirin.)

If you miss a couple of niacin doses, you may have to build up from a lower dose again to keep side effects from emerging. Be sure to let your doctor know if this happens so he can check for any effect on your cholesterol control. And ask whether you should be taking standard niacin or a slow-release niacin. Slow-release is used to avoid the sudden flood of niacin into the bloodstream and therefore decrease side effects. It can, however, be more toxic to your liver in some cases. Be sure your doctor specifies which formulation you should use.

So the emerging prognosis for niacin use seems to be this: It deserves—and is getting—a closer look from doctors and patients alike. Under a physician's supervision, niacin offers powerful help for high blood-cholesterol levels.

Gaining the Upper Hand against Disease

Arthritis: Good News   7
on the Nutrition Front

Can food defeat arthritis? Could a simple change in your diet ease the hurt? The answer used to be, "No way!" Now experts are thinking again.

It's long been known that nutrition played a big part in one type of arthritis, a painful disease called gout. Food prohibitions—no wine, beer, organ meats, or anchovies—are standard operating procedure for gout sufferers.

Firm evidence, though, just did not exist for food's role in the two major types of arthritis: rheumatoid arthritis (RA) and osteoarthritis. But scientists have uncovered the first glimmer of evidence that in some cases, dietary changes might indeed make an impact on the pain and disability of these forms of arthritis. One way that researchers think food might affect arthritis is by tinkering with the inflammation process.

Inflammation flare-ups are common in RA and are bad news because flare-ups can destroy a little more of your joints, according to Arthur I. Grayzel, M.D., senior vice-president for medical affairs for the Arthritis Foundation. So avoiding bad flare-ups may actually slow the progress of the disease.

In the latest of a series of small but well-controlled studies, researcher Joel Kremer, M.D., compared two different doses of fish oil to olive oil (a "neutral" agent) in 49 people with RA. (The fish oil contained eicosapentaenoic acid, or EPA, an omega-3 fatty acid prevalent in certain fatty fish.) After six months, signs of inflammation—pain, morning stiffness, and fatigue—improved much more in people taking the fish-oil capsules than in those taking olive oil.

And the higher dose of fish oil gave the greater improvement, says Dr. Kremer, professor of medicine at Albany Medical College, New York.

Dr. Kremer's study is his fourth on fish oil. The beneficial effects of omega-3's in people with RA have also been seen by other researchers at Harvard Medical School and Royal Adelaide Hospital in Australia.

Fish oil, a polyunsaturated fat, might help lessen inflammation, says Dr. Kremer, because it contains omega-3 fatty acids instead of omega-6 fatty acids, which are abundant in other polyunsaturated fats. Your body turns omega-6's (which are essential to health) into inflammatory chemicals called leukotrienes. Omega-3's, on the other hand, serve as alternative building blocks for biochemical products that have far less inflammatory potential.

Research like Dr. Kremer's is complicated by the "here today, gone tomorrow" nature of arthritis flare-ups. They often go away spontaneously—and stay away for long periods. (When this happens right after arthritis sufferers try some new possible remedy, they may mistakenly conclude that the remedy was responsible for the improvement.) "So some of the research subjects naturally will get better on their own, and some will get worse on their own," says Dr. Kremer. "But because we put equal numbers of all types of patients into all three groups, spontaneous improvements should happen about equally in all three and shouldn't bias one group more than the others."

So far, fish-oil researchers have focused on RA. That's because osteoarthritis is caused not by inflammation but by wearing away of cartilage (tough padding between the hard points of your bones). On the other hand, most doctors agree that osteoarthritic joints can get inflamed. The inflammation occurs when pieces of fractured cartilage break off and wedge themselves like splinters into joint linings. One small study from London did show that 26 people with osteoarthritis had less pain and freer movement after six months on fish oil. But researchers feel that fish oil's real promise is in RA.

Experts caution, though, that fish oil will never cure arthritis. For one thing, it seems to block only one of several inflammation igniters. Dr. Grayzel says fish oil may be worth a try as a supplement to medication and range-of-motion exercises, but not as a substitute.

Eating more oily fish—as often as three to five times a week—is safer than taking capsules. (Best sources of omega-3's are salmon, tuna, halibut, and sardines.) "We don't think there's any long-term danger with fish-oil capsules, but sometimes nature can fool you," says Dr. Grayzel. (Taking several spoonfuls of pure fish oil—like cod-liver oil—can be risky, too. Unlike fish-oil capsules, pure fish oil contains lots of vitamins A and D, which can be toxic in high doses.)

The Allergy Angle

Is there such a thing as "allergic arthritis"—that is, inflammation that's triggered by certain foods?

One of the few researchers doing careful, systematic investigations into allergic arthritis started out as a skeptic. He's Richard Panush, M.D., professor and chairman of the Department of Medicine at St. Barnabas Medical Center, University of Medicine and Dentistry of New Jersey. He had a patient who insisted that her arthritis acted up whenever she had milk, meat, or beans. This woman suffered from a number of sore, swollen joints and woke up each morning to a half hour of stiffness. Dr. Panush set out to determine whether she was right or wrong. First, he had her eat only a mixture containing the bare essentials of nutrition, without the alleged offending foods. After several days, her morning stiffness and joint pain disappeared.

Further evidence came when Dr. Panush gave her specially made, unmarked capsules of freeze-dried food to eat. Nothing happened after most food capsules. But after a couple capsules of freeze-dried milk powder (equivalent to an 8-ounce glass), her joints swelled and started to throb, and her morning stiffness returned full force. Her discomfort peaked 24 to 48 hours after popping the capsules. This sequence of taking milk capsules and then experiencing joint pain was repeated four times. When she was given blank capsules between these episodes, again nothing happened. Blood tests showed that her body carried milk antibodies, molecules that signal that an allergic reaction is going on. After these tests, she found that as long as she refrained from milk, she had no intense flare-ups.

Since then, 16 other patients who claimed a food/arthritis connection have undergone similar rigorous testing with Dr. Panush and his colleagues. Neither the subjects nor the researchers knew who was trying which capsules at any given time. So far, Dr. Panush has discovered three people who seem to show arthritic reactions to foods. The three include the milk case, plus a young man who reacted to shrimp, and an intensive-care nurse who reacted to nitrates, a food preservative. Subjects in Dr. Panush's experiments seem to be very special cases. Their arthritis is palindromic, which means it acts up now and then—sometimes quite severely—and then does a vanishing act. Since their joints are perfectly normal most of the time, inflammation comes on like a four-alarm fire, making it easy to record. Dr. Panush says that if allergic arthritis is real, it may affect only those with palindromic arthritis, although he doesn't rule out the possibility that some nonpalindromic arthritis may be allergic. Regardless, Dr. Panush speculates that allergic arthritis could affect only a small minority—perhaps less than 5 percent of those with rheumatoid-like arthritis.

A string of clues—some definite, some suspected—make allergic arthritis feasible, says Frederic McDuffie, M.D., arthritis center director at Piedmont Hospital, Atlanta, and former medical director of the Arthritis Foundation. First, some experts think rheumatoid arthritis allows your bowels to pass larger-than-normal food molecules through to your bloodstream. If king-size food molecules, like undigested milk protein, got into your blood, your body would take them for invaders and create antibodies to fight them. Antibodies might aggravate inflammation if they got into your joints—and we know arthritic joints let in troublemakers like inflammatory blood cells.

Experts caution that trying to identify a food allergy

without a doctor's help can be risky. Even Dr. Panush says his patients were missing certain nutrients, like calcium, while he tested them.

Compared to fish-oil research, food allergy/arthritis studies are more preliminary. And even if the evidence is borne out by larger, longer studies, only a small number of people are likely to be helped. But the potential benefit to those people is tremendous. "Here you're looking at a cause that may be constantly aggravating arthritis," says Dr. Grayzel. "Maybe if you stopped that aggravation, you would slow down the arthritis. But so far, it's still too early to say."

Dietary Changes to Make Today

While research continues on fish oil and food allergies, there's some nutritional advice that's been proven to help people with arthritis.

First, avoid obesity. David T. Felson, M.D., at the Boston University Medical School, has shown that being overweight can cause and aggravate osteoarthritis. Dr. Felson is currently testing his theory that obesity causes fluctuating hormone levels that can lead to arthritis.

Keeping weight down can be especially helpful for those who feel at risk because of a family history of arthritis and those who are in the early stages of arthritis, says Dr. Felson. But beware: Moderate weight is best. Being "pencil thin" is a major risk factor for another "osteo-." That's osteoporosis—the bodywide skeletal thinning that can be as disabling as arthritis.

Second, get more calcium (from dairy products, sardines, and leafy green vegetables) and avoid alcohol—two steps proven to fight osteoporosis. Just having arthritis puts you at greater risk for osteoporosis for three reasons. Joint inflammation breaks down nearby bones, arthritis makes it hard to do bone-strengthening exercise, and corticosteroids often prescribed for arthritis can weaken your skeleton.

Third, keep your overall nutrition at its peak. This

65
■

will help your body cope with the ups and downs of arthritis.

For more information on diet and arthritis, write to the Arthritis Foundation, P.O. Box 19000, Atlanta, GA 30326.

8 Protect Your Future by Knowing Your Past

Quick, what did your grandfather die of? What's the worst illness your aunt ever had? Does your mother take any medication? If so, for what? And what's your father's cholesterol level?

If you don't know the major illnesses and causes of death for all your siblings, parents, aunts, uncles, and grandparents, medical experts urge you to ask. It's not nosy, they say. Knowing your family medical history is crucial to your health—and the health of your children.

"Family history is second only to personal history as a guide to your medical risks," says Julie Baller, M.D., an assistant clinical professor of family and community medicine at the University of California's San Francisco Medical Center. "Once you know your family history, you can take steps to minimize your risks, and quite possibly add years to your life."

"You wouldn't think of driving across Mexico without a road map," says medical oncologist Henry Lynch, M.D., chairman of the Department of Preventive Medicine and president of the Hereditary Cancer Institute at Creighton University School of Medicine in Omaha, Nebraska. "Family medical history is a map that contains important landmarks to your health."

"Every family should compile a 'genogram,' a medical family tree," says Mack Lipkin, M.D., director of primary care and an associate professor of Medicine at Bellevue Hospital–New York Medical Center. "It takes energy, but it's very useful. Treasure it. Update it periodically. Keep it right next to the family Bible."

Unfortunately, family history is an area both patients—and physicians—may neglect. "Most doctors don't have up-to-date knowledge of hereditary factors in health," says Patricia Ward, a genetic counselor at Baylor College of Medicine in Houston. "And even when they do, it's hard to take a complete family history in the typical 15- to 20-minute office visit. That's why people need to know this information and bring it up themselves."

Which family members are important? "First- and second-degree relatives," Ward explains. "First-degree relatives are your parents, siblings, and children. Second-degree relatives are your grandparents and blood-related aunts and uncles."

What's Your Risk?

"More than 2,000 diseases run in families," Dr. Lipkin says. "Just about everyone has some family history of heart disease, cancer, and stroke, which account for more than half of U.S. deaths. The red flag is a close relative who developed any of these diseases unusually early in life. If your father died of a first heart attack at age 80, you don't have to be too concerned. But if he died at 48, then you need to take a long, hard look at your risk factors, and keep them out of the danger zone."

Alcoholism ▶ Alcohol abuse contributes to an estimated 10 percent of U.S. deaths, including those from cirrhosis, accidents, and several cancers. "Alcoholism is strongly familial," Dr. Baller says. "If any close relative is an alcoholic, I'd say don't drink. That's not easy, but in recent years it's become more socially acceptable not to."

Allergies ▶ Hay fever sometimes runs in families, Dr. Lipkin says, but polyallergy, which involves a combination of hay fever, eczema, and food sensitivities appears to be more strongly familial.

Cancer ▶ Colorectal, breast, and ovarian cancers often run in families. Colorectal cancer is the leading cancer killer among nonsmokers. One relatively rare form of the disease (familial polyposis) is strongly genetic, but many cases of colorectal cancers have inherited components. "If any first- or second-degree relative has had colorectal cancer," Dr. Lynch says, "especially if they developed it before age 50, you're at increased risk. Make sure your doctor knows your family history, and have yourself examined regularly starting in your thirties."

Breast cancer also tends to run in families. "If any first- or second-degree relative developed breast cancer before menopause, you're at considerable risk," Dr. Lynch says. "Be sure to look at your father's family as well as your mother's. If you have a family history, learn self-exam and perform it every month. Have a physician examine you regularly. And don't wait until you're 40 to start getting regular mammograms. Start having them in your twenties and thirties."

"A woman with a strong family history of breast cancer might also decide to have her first child before age 30," Dr. Baller says. "That helps reduce breast cancer risk."

Ovarian cancer is difficult to detect early and treat successfully. However, women who take birth control pills cut their risk by more than half. "The Pill has gotten a lot of bad publicity," Dr. Baller says, "but for anyone with a family history of ovarian cancer, it can be a lifesaver. You don't even have to use it that long. If you take the Pill for a few years, the protection against ovarian cancer lasts at least ten years after you stop taking it."

Cystic Fibrosis ▶ Approximately 1 child in 1,500 is born with this genetic disease, which impairs breathing and shortens life. You need two CF genes to get the disease, one from each parent. About 75 percent of people who carry one CF gene can now be identified with a blood test, Dr. Baller says. If anyone in your family—including cousins—has cystic fibrosis, consult a genetic counselor before you attempt to conceive children. (See "Do You Need Genetic Counseling?" on page 70.)

Diabetes ▶ "If one of your parents has diabetes," Dr. Lipkin says, "you have a 10 to 20 percent chance of developing it. If both parents have it, your risk rises to 50 percent." An estimated 10 million Americans have diabetes, and complications of the disease are a leading cause of death. "If you have diabetes in your family," Dr. Baller says, "that's a clear message to stay at your recommended body weight. The disease is strongly associated with obesity. Eat a low-fat diet, and get regular exercise."

Diethylstilbestrol (DES) ▶ Any woman whose mother took this hormone while pregnant is at increased risk for a rare vaginal cancer, infertility, and other medical problems. Physicians prescribed DES from the late 1940s through the 1960s in the mistaken belief that it prevented miscarriage. Tell your doctor if your mother took any prescription drugs while pregnant with you, especially if she had a history of miscarriage before you were conceived.

Ethnic Diseases ▶ Some diseases run not only in families but also in ethnic groups, Ward says. Sickle-cell disease, a potentially fatal blood disease, primarily strikes black people and those of East Indian descent. Greeks, Italians, and Asians are at risk for another potentially fatal inherited blood disorder, thalassemia. And Tay-Sachs disease, a fatal neurological disease, strikes people of French Canadian or Eastern European Jewish descent.

Heart Disease and Stroke ▶ Familial risk factors for heart disease include high cholesterol and high blood pressure (hypertension). Hypertension is also a key risk factor for stroke. "A patient of mine recently had a cholesterol test that came up 240," Dr. Baller says. "That's high, but not terribly high. Usually I'd simply recommend a low-fat diet to bring it down, but this patient's father had died fairly young of a heart attack, so we decided to treat him more aggressively, with a low-fat diet plus cholesterol-lowering medication." High blood pressure can also be reduced with a low-fat, low-salt diet, weight loss, moderate exercise, and medication.

Glaucoma ▶ Approximately one in 25 Americans develops this leading and "strongly familial" cause of blindness, Dr. Lynch says. Anyone with a family history of glaucoma should be screened regularly, because early detection and treatment can save vision.

Obesity ▶ You're "obese" if you weigh 20 percent more than the recommended weight for your height and build. "We've known for years that obesity runs in families," Dr. Lipkin says, "and recent studies have strengthened the case that it's under genetic control." Obesity is a risk factor for diabetes, hypertension, heart disease, stroke, and several cancers, including breast and colorectal. Those with a family history of obesity should work with a physician and registered dietitian to keep their weight under control.

DO YOU NEED GENETIC COUNSELING?

The answer is yes if any first- or second-degree relative has an inherited medical condition—anything from Down syndrome to cleft palate. "It's scary to face any risk of an inherited problem," says Baylor genetic counselor Patricia Ward. "But most couples assume their risk is higher than it actually is. In recent years there's been a great deal of progress in genetic screening, so we can test people for more conditions than ever. When people turn up as genetic carriers of inherited conditions, we never tell them not to have children. We help them consider their risks and options. Then they make their own decisions."

Mental Illness ▶ "Schizophrenia, depression, manic depression, and panic disorder all have genetic components," Dr. Lipkin says. "If close relatives have any of these conditions, or any history of suicide attempts, mention it to your physician, and consider psychological evaluation."

Other Diseases ▶ "For every organ system, without exception," Dr. Lipkin says, "there are diseases that run in families—kidney diseases, gastrointestinal conditions, you name it. Heart disease, cancer, stroke, diabetes, alcoholism, and mental illness are the major concerns, but the more you know about your relatives' medical history, the better."

A family history of disease in no way dooms you to serious medical problems. Nor does a robust, long-lived family guarantee you'll reach 100. "But," Dr. Baller says, "knowing your family history provides information you can use to make better-informed choices about how you live your life."

Don't Be Left Speechless 9

By Adrienne Simons

When I started my first postcollege job, I was required to screen my boss's phone calls. But each time I buzzed her over the intercom that first day, my voice sounded so strained and choked that she thought I was crying. Later that day, when I opened my mouth to say something, no sound came out. The problems continued. At the end of my first week, I was fired.

I attributed my squeezed voice to tension or the lingering effects of a cold. But when the symptoms persisted for a year, I consulted my internist. He found nothing. I saw an allergist, who thought sinusitis might be the

71

■

cause and prescribed a nasal spray. It didn't help. Finally, an otolaryngologist correctly diagnosed the problem as spasmodic, or spastic, dysphonia (SD). Like most people, I had never heard of the disorder, nor did I realize how much it would disrupt my life.

My story isn't unusual. Doctors often have trouble diagnosing SD, probably because it's fairly rare, occurring in only 5 to 10 people per 100,000. As a result, SD patients may suffer for years without a correct diagnosis. And that's too bad. Because there is hope and help for people who are diagnosed correctly.

SD is, in most cases, a form of dystonia, a movement disorder characterized by involuntary, uncontrollable muscle spasms, says Mitchell F. Brin, M.D., assistant professor of neurology at New York City's Columbia–Presbyterian Medical Center. Whereas some dystonias affect the eyelids (blepharospasm), neck (torticollis), or arm muscles (writer's cramp), SD involves spasms of the vocal cords.

Spasmodic dysphonia was described as early as 1871. Still, nearly 120 years later, the affliction continues to baffle physicians, speech experts, and patients. Because SD symptoms mimic hoarseness, physicians often misdiagnose it as laryngitis, vocal misuse, or a psychological disorder.

Doctors may refer patients for speech therapy or psychotherapy. When these treatments fail, patients may seek help through unproven techniques: hypnosis, biofeedback, acupuncture, or electroconvulsive therapy, for example. Perhaps physicians can't be faulted for their misdiagnoses and inappropriate prescriptions. Most doctors have never encountered SD. And in the absence of any visible pathology—inflamed throat, vocal cord polyps, or nodules—the doctor hears only a uniquely tight voice and concludes that the problem is vocal strain or psychological stress.

The mystery is compounded further because not all SD patients sound alike. Some voices break on almost every syllable ("My neh-Ame is Mm-Airy Jih-Owns"), while others sound gravelly. In fact, some people with SD can occasionally speak normally. And although they cannot maintain smooth speaking voices, many can laugh, cry, sigh, and yawn normally.

Anatomy of an Illness

There are actually two types of SD. The more prevalent is called adductor SD, where the voice sounds strained or strangled. Less common is abductor SD, where the person speaks in whispers.

To speak, we exhale breath through the windpipe, forcing air between the two normally closed vocal cords. The vocal cords vibrate, producing sound. When someone with adductor SD tries to talk, erratic muscle spasms lock the vocal cords together, cutting off the breath stream. As a result, the voice sounds choked. In the case of abductor SD, the vocal cords remain open and cannot vibrate properly.

Experts aren't sure what causes SD, but they do know that it's not directly caused by stress. "Stress may very well play a role at the onset of SD, however, probably by aggravating an existing imbalance in brain chemicals," says Bernadette Loftus, M.D., chief resident in otolaryngology at Columbia–Presbyterian Medical Center.

And while coping with the disorder can be emotionally stressful, the belief among experts is that SD patients are no more neurotic than people who can speak normally. "Psychotherapy may help some patients cope," says Dr. Brin, who is also coordinator of the Dystonia Clinical Research Center in New York City. "But it won't cure spasmodic dysphonia—it's a medical condition."

There is no conclusive evidence linking excessive vocal use, smoking, air pollution, or other environmental factors with SD, either.

Laryngitis is not SD. Resting your voice and drinking hot tea with honey helps to alleviate laryngitis, but not SD.

And SD is not the same as stuttering. Like SD victims, stutterers may lock their vocal cords during speech. But, unlike SD, stuttering usually begins during early childhood, and is much more prevalent among boys than girls (a 4:1 ratio). More important, though, "About 80 percent of those who stutter at one time or another spontaneously recover from it," says George H. Shames, Ph.D., professor of communication disorders and psychology at the University of Pittsburgh. Spontaneous recovery from SD is exceedingly rare.

The People with SD

Experts can't pinpoint precisely how many people suffer from SD, partly because so many patients are misdiagnosed. Many SD patients who attribute a strained voice to "nerves" never seek medical attention at all. And since SD patients often consult more than one specialist, it's difficult to maintain an accurate count. "We just don't know if we're all treating different cases or the same people," says Carole S. Bloch, a speech pathologist and consultant to New York Hospital–Cornell Medical Center in New York City.

Researchers, however, have developed a demographic profile of SD patients. "It's 1½ times more common in women than in men," says Dr. Loftus. The average age of onset is about 35; most patients are between 30 and 60.

After reviewing many patients' family trees, Dr. Brin believes SD may have a genetic link. In fact, he and other leading SD researchers believe "it is of paramount importance to get the patient's family history [and] provide genetic counseling," so SD patients can learn what the potential is to pass this on to their offspring.

Whoever they are, SD patients are likely to suffer the same frustrations. Perhaps ordinary situations best epitomize the experience of SD. Just about everything that most other people do without thinking becomes a potential snag: asking for help in a store, ordering a meal in a restaurant, calling for a haircut appointment, introducing yourself.

Aside from these everyday problems, SD can also disrupt your social life. Charles, 47, has SD and finds it "very difficult to form new friendships. After a while, I became somewhat paranoid about approaching people," he says.

"I have lost many friends," laments Bernice, 40. "People do not call me back when I leave a shaky-voiced message on their answering machine."

Gatherings cause anxiety between SD sufferers and their spouses. Forty-seven-year-old Betty confesses, "I avoided parties my husband wanted to go to, avoided inviting people to my home, and avoided calling friends." Telephones are a constant nemesis because the only way to communicate over the phone is with your voice.

People with SD often avoid public speaking, too. I recall leading a prayer in synagogue. Afterward, congregation members asked me why I was crying. I quickly claimed I had laryngitis.

And imagine your voice forcing a career change! Charles left his career as an employment counselor to work in a warehouse. Ironically, a speech pathologist with SD works only with deaf clients, using sign language.

Relief and Comfort

If you suspect you have SD, you should visit an otolaryngologist (ear, nose, and throat specialist). He can examine your larynx (upper windpipe) with a small mirror and with a fiberoptic endoscope inserted through a nostril. Using both methods, he inspects the vocal cords for structural abnormalities and observes their activity during speech.

A neurologist should also examine you to reveal or rule out any other neurological disorder.

And you should see a speech pathologist, whose trained ear evaluates voice quality. The diagnosis should be based on the findings of all three specialists.

After a diagnosis is nailed down, you can get the help you need. Voice therapy with an experienced speech pathologist (one who has worked with SD patients) teaches new methods of breathing and voicing. Using these tech-

75

niques, some patients are able to reduce the tight spasticity in their voice. The long-term success rate is low, however, so many SD patients are prompted to seek medical alternatives.

One such treatment is the surgical "laryngeal nerve section." Developed in the mid-1970s, this involves severing the laryngeal nerve, which paralyzes one vocal cord and helps reduce muscle spasms. The success rate is only about 30 percent after three years, however.

A new, highly reliable treatment involves injecting very tiny amounts of botulinum toxin (nicknamed "Botox") directly into the laryngeal muscle. Botox "chemically paralyzes the laryngeal muscle by blocking the release of the neurotransmitter acetylcholine from the laryngeal nerve," says Dr. Brin, whose research team pioneered the treatment. As a result, the vocal spasms are reduced and the voice sounds more normal. Botox is approved by the Food and Drug Administration for treatment of facial dystonia, but not yet approved specifically for SD. Physicians are permitted to use it for this purpose, however, although only a few specialists currently have expertise in this area.

Researcher Christy Ludlow, Ph.D., at the National Institutes of Health in Bethesda, Maryland, reports significant improvements in 148 of 150 SD patients receiving Botox treatment. Dr. Brin reports success in all 275 patients he has treated this way.

Botox produces a fairly normal voice for two to four months, when another injection is needed. Considering how many patients have suffered in silence, Botox seems like a miracle drug. However, Botox is a toxic substance and no long-term studies have yet been conducted with SD patients. (In facial dystonia patients, it can cause atrophy of facial muscle, which may be partly reversible.)

If you have SD, the best approach is to learn everything you can about each treatment, then choose the one you're most comfortable with. Treatment may be only part of the answer, though.

In coping with SD, it can be very helpful to meet with other patients. There are 28 support groups in the

United States and 3 in Canada. These groups are sponsored by local hospitals or research centers.

Midge Kovacs, managing editor of the national SD newsletter, "Our Voice," and founder of the New York City support group, recalls the 1987 birth of her group: "Fifteen people attended our first meeting. There was a lot of crying because no one had ever met another SD patient before." Since then, her group's mailing list has grown to 156. She is convinced that fear, anxiety, confusion over treatment options, and lack of information prompt patients to join the groups.

In addition to providing emotional support, these groups share medical literature, hold coping workshops (where they learn telephone coping tips, stress reduction, and job interview techniques, for example), and invite experts to discuss the latest research results.

In 1990, the National Spasmodic Dysphonia Association (NSDA) was established to help educate the public, promote research, and encourage the formation of support groups.

For more information on SD, send a self-addressed, stamped envelope to the NSDA at P.O. Box 266, Birmingham, MI 48012, or the Dystonia Medical Research Foundation, 8383 Wilshire Boulevard, Suite 800, Beverly Hills, CA 90211. For a copy of "Our Voice," send a self-addressed, stamped envelope to: Our Voice, 799 Broadway, Suite 640, New York, NY 10003.

Children and Cancer   10
Prevention

There are lots of things adults can do to decrease their cancer risks, and, although you don't hear much about it, there are things you can do to reduce your children's lifetime cancer risks as well. The latest research and best medical minds in the country agree: One of the most important gifts you can give a child is an edge against the risks for cancer. Here are the recommendations for prudent action now.

Clear the Air

Most parents would have a fit if they saw their child smoking. Even parents who smoke don't want their children to pick up the habit. Yet smokers are putting their children at greater risk for cancer, whether the kids follow in their footsteps or not.

The problem is called "passive smoking"—exposure to tobacco smoke from others in enclosed, poorly ventilated spaces—an issue that's gotten a lot of press in the past few years. Many studies have examined the cancer risks of nonsmokers who are married to smokers. But one of the latest studies looks specifically at childhood exposure to "secondhand" smoke.

Since lung cancer is rare in nonsmokers, the researchers rounded up 191 people who had never smoked and yet had the disease. Passive smoke exposure was determined by the number of years spent in each residence multiplied by the number of smokers living there concurrently. (One year of living with one smoker is called one "smoker year.") An equal number of nonsmokers without lung cancer were interviewed and asked to serve as a control group.

The results: Exposure to 25 or more smoker years during childhood and adolescence doubled the risk of lung cancer in nonsmoking adults. "That means if both the child's parents smoke, that child has twice the risk of developing lung cancer by age 12 or 13 as kids who have nonsmoking parents," warns Martin F. McKneally, M.D., one of the authors of the study and chief of thoracic surgery at University of Toronto General Hospital. The more smokers in the house, the quicker the damage is done to young lungs. "Passive smoking should be a real concern, especially if there's a history of cancer in the family," Dr. McKneally says.

So the experts are unanimous in their advice: Don't

expose your children to your smoke. And just as important: Don't let your child start using tobacco in any form—including snuff or chewing tobacco, which is popular with preteen boys. Some teenagers who are long-time snuff users have been disfigured by severe cases of oral cancer.

Avoid Toxic Exposure

Exposure to insecticides and weedkillers at home has been linked to increased risk of various types of cancer in children and adults. One of the more alarming reports found that either parent's use of household insecticides during the mother's pregnancy increased the child's normally low risk of leukemia nearly fourfold. (For white children, that's a jump from a 1 in 1,610 risk to about 1 in 403; for blacks, a 1 in 2,730 risk becomes 1 in 683.) The same study found that either parent's use of garden insecticides and weedkillers during the mother's pregnancy multiplied childhood leukemia risks 6½ times above average.

The level of chemical use associated with these risks is high: at least once a week indoors; at least once a month with the stronger outdoor varieties. Childhood leukemia is a relatively rare disease, and the increased risks don't translate into an overwhelming number of cases. But for a risk that's so easily avoided, it makes sense for a parent to take every precaution.

"It seems reasonable to assume that parents continued using insecticides at the same rate after the child was born," says John M. Peters, M.D., professor of preventive medicine at the University of Southern California. "We're currently working on a follow-up study that tracks the child's exposure to these toxic substances."

"The main concern about childhood chemical exposure is that we don't know enough about the long-term effects," says Shiela H. Zahm, Sc.D., an epidemiologist at the National Cancer Institute. For example, two of Dr. Zahm's studies tracked an increased risk of lymphoma (cancer of the lymph glands) in farmers using a weed-killer known as 2,4-D (2,4-dichlorophenoxyacetic acid). "This substance is an active ingredient in several over-the-counter lawn and garden sprays, and it's still used by most lawn-care companies," Dr. Zahm says. "We studied farmers, so we don't know what the risk is to children who live in households where 2,4-D is used on the lawns. There is reason for concern, however, because for some chemicals, children tend to be more sensitive than adults are."

The best course of action for your household? Limit or eliminate insecticides and weedkillers whenever possible. Doing so can lower your child's cancer risks now and as an adult. But if you choose to use these substances, you should take the following precautions.

Keep Kids out of the Yard ▶ Not just during application of weedkillers and insecticides, but after, too. "If you spray your lawn, as a precaution don't let children play in the yard for three days," says Dr. Zahm.

Ventilate the House ▶ "After using a whole-room insecticide, like flea or roach bombs, ventilate with open windows and fans for at least 4 or 5 hours to remove toxic levels from the air," warns Richard Fenske, Ph.D., associate professor of environmental health at the University of Washington, Seattle.

Keep Infants and Toddlers off the Floor ▶ And any other surface where insecticides have been sprayed for at least 24 hours after application.

Use Traps instead of Sprays ▶ "Ant and roach traps are much more efficient and less hazardous to humans than sprays," says Dr. Fenske. As long as children can't get at the poison, traps are preferable.

Reduce Radiation Risks

Exposure to high doses of radiation is a known cancer risk, but not all sources of radiation are equally risky.

Radon, a naturally occurring gas that's released by radioactive particles in the soil, has been dubbed the second most important cause of lung cancer by the Environmental Protection Agency (EPA). But the EPA's pronouncement is based primarily on data from miners exposed to radon underground. Can data from miners spell a risk to minors? "There's just not enough evidence to determine the real risk of radon in the home," says Edward Trapido, Sc.D., an epidemiologist at the University of Miami School of Medicine.

The prudent advice seems to be: Have the radon levels in your home tested. If they are significantly higher than the EPA's guidelines, you may want to take steps to vent the gas out of your house. Remember: While the greatest radon concentration is usually in the basement, you should have the rooms in which your family spends a lot of time tested, like bedrooms and the family room.

The amount of risk from electromagnetic radiation is also controversial and very speculative at this point. There's no conclusive evidence that fields in power tools, electric blankets, appliances, and electrical wiring pose a health threat. (The majority of experts rate electromagnetic radiation extremely low as a risk for cancer.) The possibility of electromagnetic fields being a health risk wasn't raised until 1979, when a study in Denver found children who had died from leukemia and other cancers were more likely to have lived near ordinary neighborhood power lines that carry a higher than average current.

There have been many subsequent studies looking at various types of electromagnetic-field exposure. Some found no significant correlation with cancer risks. Others, including studies of high occupational exposure in power company linemen, found some elevated risk of cancer. One preliminary study claims that kids exposed to strong electromagnetic fields appear to have a slightly increased risk of developing certain cancers. Normal risk of getting cancer is 1 in 10,000; the exposed children's risk was 2 in 10,000. Several major studies are trying to confirm this finding.

The bottom line: The real risk, if any, is hard to weigh based on the evidence so far, but it can't hurt to be cautious regarding power lines. Any significant risk comes from long-term exposure, so don't let children play directly under power lines. That goes for regular lines as well as high-tension wires. The electromagnetic field drops off rapidly as you move out from under them.

And what about radiation from home computers, TVs, and video games? "As long as the child doesn't spend a lot of time right on top of the screen, there's not much to worry about. The electromagnetic field tends to be greater at the back of these machines than the front," says David O. Carpenter, M.D., dean of the School of Public Health at the State University of New York at Albany.

The type of radiation used in diagnostic x-rays can increase cancer risks by a very small amount as exposures are repeated over the years. But the difference between x-rays and most other sources of radiation is that the x-ray is done for some medical benefit. "The information gained is worth the tiny exposure involved when used with good medical judgment," says David F. Adcock, M.D., chairman of radiology at the University of South Carolina at Columbia.

Except for the odd broken bone, the most x-ray exposure to children takes place at the dentist's office. The exposure for an individual picture is very low. Although x-rays are relatively safe, there are still a few precautions the concerned parent can take.

Be Sure the Lead Apron Covers the Neck ▶ "The thyroid gland, which sits over the windpipe in the neck, is very sensitive to radiation, especially in children. In general, the younger the child the more sensitive he or she will be. Covering the child's neck during dental x-rays decreases the risk of radiation-induced thyroid cancer," says Dr. Adcock.

Keep a Record of X-rays ▶ The greater the radiation exposure over a lifetime, the greater the risk of any radiation-induced cancer. It's not a bad idea to keep a record of the type and number of x-rays your child undergoes. That way, your child's physician can make an informed decision about an individual x-ray examination.

There's no magic level of radiation that would be considered too much for medical purposes, but there should be no radiation exposure that doesn't provide useful diagnostic information.

Shade Out Excess Sun

Parents tend to forget about the most important source of radiation exposure: ultraviolet radiation from the sun. "Kids are outside more than you'd think—far more than many adults," says John J. DiGiovanna, M.D., a dermatologist at the National Cancer Institute. "And sun exposure is the primary cause of skin cancer."

The risks of skin cancer from excess sun are twofold: (1) Just one bad sunburn can increase your child's chances of developing malignant melanoma, the most serious kind of skin cancer, later in life. People can die from melanomas that aren't treated in time. (2) Frequent sun exposure can raise your child's risk of developing basal-cell and squamous-cell carcinomas. Even without causing a burn, long-term sun exposure can damage cells enough to trigger these more easily treated forms of skin cancer.

"A child's skin is thinner and has less protective melanin (the pigment that goes into freckles and tans) than an adult's skin. So children need more protection from the sun than their parents do," Dr. DiGiovanna advises.

Keep Infants Covered ▶ Start babies off right by shading them from strong sunlight. Bonnets, hats, covered carriages, and strollers are the best outdoor protection the little nipper has. Protective clothing is a good idea for older kids, too.

Slather on Sunscreen ▶ Beyond the baby stage, it's hard to keep kids out of the sun. But you can shield them with sunscreen with a high sun protection factor (SPF).

SPF-15 is good. Mom or Dad should apply the sunscreen to make sure smaller children are covered adequately over all exposed areas. And reapply the sunscreen if it's washed off by water or perspiration.

Limit Sun Time during Peak Hours ▶ Ultraviolet rays are strongest between 10:00 A.M. and 3:00 P.M. When at a place with little shade—the beach, for example—it would be wise to limit your child's noontime fun-in-the-sun activities. At home, parents can set up play areas, swings, and sandboxes in shady parts of the yard.

Obviously, lighter-skinned families need to be more careful. But even blacks can get skin cancer (although it's much, much rarer than in whites). For that reason, black children shouldn't get excessive amounts of sun exposure either, and light-skinned blacks ought to use sunscreen.

Feed Them Right

There's a great deal of good evidence that a healthy, balanced diet can lower cancer rates in adults. And experts believe that this applies no less to children. Even though kids tend to be pickier eaters than their parents, there are two simple ways to improve their diet.

Reduce Fat in the Diet ▶ With the kinds of things kids like to eat, this is easier said than done. "But it's a worthwhile measure, since there's an association between high fat intake and certain cancers in adults. Besides, a diet in which less than 30 percent of calories come from fat has other health benefits as well," says Alice S. Bennett, Ph.D., professor of biology at Ball State University.

A caution, however: Don't try to restrict fat in the diet of children under age two. They need a higher ratio of fat for proper growth and nutrition.

Serve Lots of Fruit and/or Vegetables ▶ Children should have at least five servings daily. There is strong evidence from dozens of population studies that a high intake of fruits and veggies leads to reduced cancer risks.

"It's not as hard as it sounds to get five servings in," says Gladys Block, Ph.D., of the National Cancer Institute. "A glass of fruit juice at breakfast, a piece of fruit with lunch, another as a snack, and two vegetables with dinner will do it. And since kids tend to like fruits and salads more than vegetables, it's okay to substitute with these at dinner if the kids won't eat their veggies then."

And what about pesticide residues on fruits and vegetables? "I feel that the bigger risk comes when children do not eat these foods each day," Dr. Block says.

"There are no reported cases of cancer that have been linked to legal use of pesticides in the United States," says Susan Foerester, chief of nutrition and cancer prevention at the California Health Department. "Only about 12 percent of the produce tested has detectable amounts of residue. And what is found is very minimal and well below legal safety margins."

Whip High Blood Pressure with a Workout   11

Rarely does news this good come out about a problem so bad: The new treatment for high blood pressure has finally arrived. After years of scientific testing, it's made the grade and become the potent Third Option—beyond drugs and diet. But it has some strange side effects: It can make you feel younger, and look younger, too. It can increase blood levels of HDL cholesterol (the beneficial type), help you lose weight, decrease stress, and lower risk of heart disease. It's also as natural as a sunset and as easy as a walk in the park. And it's free.

It's exercise.

For years research has been slowly piling up to show that regular workouts may lower blood pressure by 5 to 20 points. But now two studies appear to give the final blessing to the Third Option—by suggesting that it may have far more power to lower blood pressure, and do it in more interesting ways, than anyone thought.

"Results of this research could substantially change the way we treat moderate and borderline cases of this very serious problem," says hypertension researcher John Martin, Ph.D., of San Diego State University. "Exercise seems to work more directly in lowering blood pressure than previously had been thought."

Gain without Loss

In one of the new studies, Dr. Martin and his colleagues put 19 sedentary men with mild hypertension through either an aerobic exercise program or a "placebo" regimen (slow calisthenics and stretching). After ten weeks, the blood pressure of the men in the aerobic group dropped dramatically—from an average of 137/95 at the beginning of the study to 130/85 at the end. That's a change from mild hypertension to high-normal blood pressure. "These drops were significant because they brought our test subjects' readings down out of the range where drug therapy often is considered," Dr. Martin says. The placebo group, on the other hand, actually had a slight increase in blood pressure. And later, when they were placed on the exercise program, they showed similar reductions in blood pressure.

This big improvement in the exercisers was expected, but something else was a pleasant surprise. "Scientists have known for years that losing weight could lower blood pressure," Dr. Martin says. "And they thought that exercise could lower blood pressure only if it also produced substantial weight loss. But that appears not to be the case. Our study found significant blood pressure reductions even though participants did not experience sizable decreases in weight or body fat."

If these findings are borne out by other research, it will mean that exercise has not one but two mechanisms for beating mild hypertension.

Then there was something else. Previous research

suggested that it was vigorous exercise that brought blood pressure down. But in this study the subjects weren't exercising strenuously enough to make profound gains in aerobic endurance. Despite that fact, significant reductions in blood pressure still occurred. Diastolic blood pressure (the second number, which measures arterial pressure while the heart is at rest) came down by an average of 9.6 points, and systolic pressure (the measurement of pressure as the heart contracts) fell by 6.4 points.

"People in our study exercised at levels well within their comfort zone. Their exercise consisted of either walking, cycling, or jogging, or doing any combination of these activities for approximately 30 minutes, four times a week," says Dr. Martin. "The subsequent reduction in blood pressure suggests that physical activity of even fairly light intensity may be more helpful against hypertension than previous research has led us to think."

None of this means, though, that reducing body fat and increasing aerobic fitness are not advisable antihypertensive strategies. "Our research simply suggests that exercise may have valuable effects in normalizing blood pressure that work independently of these two other mechanisms," Dr. Martin says.

Workouts vs. Wonder Drugs

The other study was conducted at the Columbia Medical Plan, Columbia, Maryland, in conjunction with Johns Hopkins School of Medicine. In it 52 men between ages 18 and 59 with mild hypertension were asked to exercise regularly for ten weeks while taking either blood pressure medication or a placebo (inactive pill). Sure enough, blood pressure dropped in all the subjects (including those who didn't take medication) from an average of 145/97 to 131/84. Again this decrease was reached without substantial weight loss. The real news here, however, was that the data suggest that aerobic exercise may not be the only kind of workout that can help lower blood pressure. Three days a week, for 50 minutes per workout, the participants in this study walked/jogged or rode a stationary bike and—surprisingly enough—did weight training. It's surprising because weight training tends to raise blood pressure during the actual lifting and so has long been considered too risky an exercise for people with high blood pressure.

"The findings suggest that weight training need not be dangerous if the lifting is kept fairly light," says one of the researchers, Mark Effron, M.D., of Sinai Hospital in Baltimore. "All of the lifts in our study were performed at 40 percent of a participant's maximal capability, which is a level reported to be associated with acceptable rises

BORDERLINE HYPERTENSION MORE DANGEROUS THAN EXPECTED

So exercise can wrestle down blood pressure naturally, and with no side effects other than greater energy, a firmer physique, and a shot in the arm for self-esteem. It's great news.

But the news becomes even greater in light of an important discovery from researchers at the University of Michigan Hospitals in Ann Arbor. They found that borderline hypertension—either 140 to 1f9 systolic (the first number) or 90 to 95 diastolic—appears to pose greater risks to the cardiovascular system than previously had been thought. A random sampling of 946 people between the ages of 18 and 38 found that those whose blood pressure was in the borderline range (approximately 12 percent of the total group) had significantly greater cardiovascular abnormalities than the people whose pressure was normal.

Levels of total cholesterol, triglycerides, and in-

in blood pressure." The weight training was done for 30 minutes each session in a circuit fashion, where lifts were done on 20 different variable-resistance machines.

"While we did find that blood pressure was elevated more just after weight training than after the aerobic exercise," says Dr. Effron, "the difference in measurement was only slight."

"What's more, pulse rates were lower during the weight training than during the aerobic activities, so the overall demands being put on the heart by the two types of exercise proved to be roughly the same. That's a significant finding. And it's very encouraging news for the strength-conscious."

sulin all were higher, while HDL cholesterol (the good kind) was lower in the borderline group. The borderline group also showed signs of having less flexible arteries than the normal group, and their hearts showed signs of having lost elasticity and hence pumping power.

"We used to think of borderline hypertension as a gray area, but we now have reason to believe it's darker than we had thought," says study director Steve Julius, M.D. "People with borderline hypertension are likely to be at a significantly greater risk for suffering from cardiovascular disease than people whose pressures are normal. They should make concentrated efforts through exercise, weight control, and restriction of sodium, dietary fat, tobacco, and alcohol to bring their pressures down. Only if these strategies fail should pharmacologic [drug] treatment be considered."

Also significant in this study was the discovery that blood pressure drugs administered in addition to exercise did not lower blood pressure any more than exercise alone. "Patients engaged in a regular program of exercise may not need drug therapy for control of mild hypertension," the authors of the study conclude. That's big news for the estimated 40 million Americans with blood pressure readings in the moderately high range (a diastolic pressure of 90 or more). Not all these people could do without medication, but moderate workouts could help many of them get off their drugs or not have to use drugs in the first place.

"They should get complete medical clearance from their doctors first, of course, but if an exercise program is approached sensibly, it can be a highly recommendable option to standard drug therapy," Dr. Effron says.

One more interesting piece of evidence uncovered in the study: Although both exercise and the drugs lowered blood pressure equally well, exercise alone actually proved superior to one of the drugs (propranolol) in affecting cholesterol. Exercise lowered total blood cholesterol and low-density lipoprotein (LDL) cholesterol (the heart-clogging kind) and raised high-density lipoprotein (HDL) cholesterol (the beneficial type). This has been demonstrated in other research, too. But in this study, propranolol lowered HDL, which might be a disadvantage for anyone concerned about heart disease.

The Whys of Success

So why is it that high blood pressure yields to a little human muscle? Why should firming up the muscles help loosen up the arteries? You might think just the opposite would be true.

"We're not sure yet, but there are some theories," Dr. Martin says. "It may well be that the amount of inactivity many of us have been accustomed to is simply unnatural from a biological standpoint. A certain level of physical movement may be necessary to keep the body's blood pressure–regulating mechanisms working the way they should.

"We know, for example, that small arteries can begin to shut down through lack of physical activity, and that regulatory hormones from the kidneys can be adversely affected. Add the effects of psychological stress that can result from too sedentary a lifestyle and you can begin to see just how extensive the ill effects of too little activity can be."

So if you have high blood pressure and you've been given a green light by your doctor, there's no reason not to take your condition "by the horns and wrestle it to the ground" with a sensible and moderate exercise program. Try to do something, even if it's just going for a walk or doing yard chores for about 30 minutes at least three days a week.

In combination with whatever other blood pressure–beating tactics you can employ (i.e., cutting back on sodium, alcohol, tobacco, and stress), you should be able to give your blood pressure a darned good run for its money.

Optimal Aging

Update on Osteoporosis   12

What can you do—starting today—to forestall osteoporosis, the disease of fragile and porous bones that afflicts 24 million Americans? And what can you do tomorrow—in the other stages of your life—to keep up the good fight?

You can do plenty. There are some very positive preventive (and treatment) strategies right at your fingertips—from calcium intake to bone-strengthening exercise to bone-building drugs and experimental treatments.

And this is your guide to all of them: what you can do, how to do it, and what it'll do for your bones at each time of your life.

Bad to the Bone

Did you ever have a child ask you, "How come I have to drink milk when you get to have soda?" If your answer was the classic, "Your bones are still growing—mine aren't," you weren't quite telling the truth. In fact, bone tissue in both children and adults is constantly "turning over." That is, minerals like calcium are continually being deposited and removed.

During childhood and adolescence, deposits exceed withdrawals as new bone is added to the skeleton. The result: heavier, denser bones. This goes on until somewhere between the ages of 25 and 35, when your bones attain what experts call "peak bone mass." You'll never have more bone than this for the rest of your life.

No matter what your peak bone mass (the amount of bone tissue you have) is, from about age 35 on, women and men begin to slowly lose bone as the withdrawals of minerals exceed deposits.

Osteoporosis is an exaggerated loss of bone tissue that usually begins developing in women after menopause, when the body produces much less estrogen (a hormone that helps protect bones). This stepped-up rate of bone loss usually occurs ten years or more later in men.

At any stage of adulthood, osteoporosis can also be a side effect of certain medications, including glucocorticoids, thyroid hormone, and antiseizure drugs. It's important for people on these drugs to ask their physicians to monitor them for osteoporosis. Cigarette smoking and excessive alcohol intake are risk factors for bone loss as well.

If you lose too much bone tissue, the result can be weaker bones that are prone to fracture. And fractures are serious business. Osteoporosis alone is responsible for 1.3 million broken bones each year—most commonly in the wrist, hip, and spinal vertebrae.

When you have osteoporosis, you don't have to fall hard to break a bone. Seemingly mundane activities of everyday life, such as bending over to pet your dog or to pick up a light package, may be all it takes.

Hip fractures, which occur four times more often in women than in men, can lead to fatality as much as 20 percent of the time. That's hard to believe, but complications such as pneumonia or blood clots in the lungs can be related to the fracture itself or to surgery. About one out of four people who break a hip after the age of 55 will not be able to walk again without help. And crushed and weakened vertebrae can lead to shrunken height, curvature of the spine, and back pain.

But the good news, according to William A. Peck, M.D., founding president of the National Osteoporosis Foundation (NOF), is that "osteoporosis need not be an inevitable part of aging." It's never too late to take preventive steps. True, prevention of bone loss is more effective in the early stages of osteoporosis, but it's important to stop further losses in people who already have a more advanced problem.

Strategy 1: Calcium

Experts agree that lifelong intake of adequate calcium is your best hedge against osteoporosis. (Yet it's estimated that a third of middle-aged and elderly women consume less than 400 milligrams of calcium a day—far short of their needs.)

The controversial issue: Does calcium—whether from foods or supplements—help prevent bone loss after menopause? Studies have yielded conflicting results. Yet, according to Robert Heaney, M.D., chairman of Congress's Office of Technology Assessment's scientific advisory panel on osteoporosis, bone mass per se is less important than fractures. "And in preventing fractures," he says, "the evidence for calcium is strong."

In one study, women whose lifetime dietary calcium intake was about 1,000 milligrams per day had 60 to 75 percent fewer hip fractures than women consuming around 500 milligrams. Another study showed that both men and women over 60 years old who daily consumed more than 765 milligrams of calcium had a hip fracture rate that was 60 percent lower than people who got less than 470 milligrams.

British authors have estimated that "If calcium were only 1 percent more effective than a placebo in reducing the incidence of fractures, it may be able to prevent more than 1,000 fractures a year in Britain." Our conclusion: Consuming adequate calcium throughout your life is very important for strong, healthy bones, even if you start today. The reality is that—whether you're young or old—if you don't consume enough of the mineral, your body will take calcium from your bones to make it available for life-sustaining activities, such as nerve conduction, muscle contraction, and blood clotting. So how much calcium should you consume—and at what times of your life? Here's our best advice, based on the evidence.

Childhood and Early Adulthood ▶ Many experts now believe that the best nutritional way to lower the risk of osteoporosis in later life is to ensure the adequate intake of calcium when the bone's peak mass is being accumulated. The key time is throughout childhood up to the age of 35.

According to Charles W. Slemenda, D.P.H., from the Department of Medicine at the Indiana University School of Medicine, adults with the highest calcium intakes as children and adolescents seem to have about 5 percent more bone than those with the lowest intakes. The larger your peak bone mass, the more resistant you probably are to osteoporosis and the lower your risk of fractures at any age.

For children between the ages of 1 and 10, we recommend a daily calcium intake of 800 milligrams; from 11 to 24, 1,200 milligrams; and from 25 to 35, 800 to 1,000 milligrams. Pregnant or lactating women should get 1,200 to 1,600 milligrams a day.

The Thirties and Forties ▶ "The idea for women is to go into menopause with as much bone as possible," says Dr. Heaney, "because calcium won't help as much right after they stop menstruating." And preliminary evidence suggests that consuming plenty of calcium-rich foods the decade or so before menopause (which typically occurs around the age of 50) may indeed make a crucial difference to bone strength later on.

Daniel T. Baran, M.D., and his colleagues at the University of Massachusetts Medical Center, found that 30- to 40-year-old women who consumed 1,500 milligrams of calcium daily from low-fat, calcium-rich foods had lost none of their bone mass over three years, while women who got just 800 milligrams of calcium a day lost 3 percent of their bone. According to Dr. Baran, that significant difference might translate into having 20 to 30 percent more bone by the time the high-calcium consumers reach menopause.

The best advice for premenopausal women: Consume 1,000 milligrams of calcium a day.

Around Menopause ▶ The truth is that no amount of calcium alone can totally overcome the loss of bone that occurs during early menopause. However, in several well-designed studies of calcium supplementation in perimenopausal (around the time of menopause) women, modest increases in bone mass occurred. Another benefit of calcium is that it may lower the effective dose of estrogen needed to prevent bone loss. In one study it was found that postmenopausal women who took a 1,000-milligram calcium supplement were able to take half the usual dose of estrogen therapy to achieve the same effect as a full dose of estrogen in women who didn't take calcium.

The best advice: Consume 1,000 milligrams of calcium daily if you're on estrogen and 1,500 milligrams if you're not.

65 and Older ▶ By ages 65 to 70, women and men lose bone at the same rate. Although increasing calcium intake alone cannot prevent or reverse osteoporosis in the elderly, Dr. Heaney believes that calcium is at least as important at this time as before menopause. In part, it's because both men and women are less efficient at absorbing calcium as they age.

The best advice: Consume between 1,000 and 1,500 milligrams a day.

Getting Your Calcium ▶ Most experts agree that the best way to get your calcium is from foods. The best sources are milk products, including low-fat and skim milk, buttermilk, and low-fat yogurt and cheese. Broccoli and collard, kale, and turnip greens are also rich in calcium, as are fish like canned salmon and mackerel when bones and all are eaten. (See "Calcium Reminders: Ways to Put More in Your Diet" on page 98.)

Yet for women who can't or don't get enough calcium from foods, "there is definitely a place for calcium supplements," says NOF board member John Renner, M.D. But supplements should complement—not take the place of—food sources of calcium. To make sure you're getting the appropriate amount of calcium from supplements, you need to guesstimate how much you're getting from your food. (Check food labels for calcium content.) Together, the calcium you get from food and the amount you get from supplements should come close to your total recommended calcium level.

How much calcium is too much? If you consume more than 2,500 milligrams a day, you might excrete too much calcium in your urine, a potential hazard for someone prone to developing kidney stones. So check with your

CALCIUM REMINDERS: WAYS TO PUT MORE IN YOUR DIET

Whole-milk dairy products have a lot of calcium, but they also have a fair amount of fat, and much of it is saturated. Here are some heart-healthy calcium alternatives.

• Whenever possible, substitute skim or low-fat milk for water—for example, in soup, oatmeal, and muffins.

• Have broccoli, collard, kale, or turnip greens several times a week. (Spinach contains a lot of calcium, too, but it also has substances called oxalates that interfere with its absorption.)

• Add several heaping spoonfuls of nonfat dry milk to anything you can think of—meat loaf, casseroles, soups, and beverages. (Nonfat dry milk, when stirred into coffee, tastes and looks like half-and-half.)

• Eat more low-fat yogurt and frozen yogurt in place of conventional desserts. (Remember though:

physician before beginning a high-calcium regimen—particularly if you have a family history of kidney stones. It's also wise to drink lots of water—about six to eight 8-ounce glasses a day—if you're taking a calcium supplement.

When you take your calcium supplements is important, too. Studies suggest that they're best absorbed when taken in divided doses, throughout the day—and if you take them with meals. In one study, just two 250-milligram doses of calcium provided more absorbable calcium than one 1,000-milligram dose.

On an ounce-for-ounce basis, yogurt has at least as much calcium as milk, but it's not generally fortified with vitamin D as milk is.)

• Grate low-fat cheese over salads, soups, and casseroles. (Note that cottage cheese is not a particularly good source of calcium, and low-calcium cream cheese is largely fat.)

• Try tofu (soybean curd); use it in place of meat or chicken in favorite stir-fry recipes or add it to soups and salads. (Check the label to make sure the tofu was processed with a calcium salt. Four ounces can have as much as 300 milligrams of calcium.)

• Have low-fat milk shakes instead of soft drinks—mix milk, ice cubes, flavoring, and low-cal sweetener in a blender.

• Snack on broccoli with dips made from plain yogurt or part-skim ricotta cheese.

Strategy 2: Vitamin D

If you get your calcium from a source other than dairy products, you may miss out on vitamin D, a nutrient added to most milk in the United States. And what does vitamin D intake have to do with osteoporosis?

Vitamin D is necessary for the body to use calcium. If you're deficient, your body can't absorb calcium adequately from the diet. So it pulls calcium from your bones to maintain blood levels. "Eventually, you can develop a defect in the bone mineralization process, which accelerates osteoporosis," says Michael Holick, M.D., Ph.D., director of the Vitamin D and Bone Research Laboratory at Boston University School of Medicine. "In Boston, we're finding that between 30 and 40 percent of hip fracture patients are vitamin D–deficient."

Of course, the body can make its own vitamin D when the skin is exposed to sunlight. But with warnings to stay out of the sun because of skin cancer risk, many of us are limiting our doses of sunshine.

Our recommendations:

Young to Middle-Aged People ▶ If you're reasonably active outdoors—getting casual exposure to sunlight—then you don't need to worry about vitamin D. Calcium should be your main concern. Even though the sun is at the wrong angle to allow your skin to make vitamin D in the winter, your body can draw upon stores in fat tissue.

If you rarely go outdoors, rest assured that just 2 cups of fortified skim, low-fat, or whole milk a day can provide you with the adult Recommended Dietary Allowance (RDA) of 200 international units of vitamin D. Some cereals are fortified with the vitamin, too. You can also get substantial amounts of vitamin D from oilier types of fish, such as mackerel, salmon, and herring.

Older Men and Women ▶ As we age, skin is less efficient at making the sunshine vitamin. Not only that, but older people are less efficient at converting vitamin

D from foods and supplements to a usable form. In an article in the *American Journal of Clinical Nutrition,* Dr. Holick and his co-workers reported on findings that in a group of more than 180 elderly people, 70 to 80 percent of them were borderline to overtly vitamin D–deficient in the wintertime. But people taking a 400-international unit vitamin D supplement had no problems.

So Dr. Holick thinks it's especially important for people who are 65-plus to make a special effort to either drink 2 cups of milk or to spend a little time in the sun. Dr. Holick's advice is to go out in the sun for 5 to 10 minutes (with face, arms, and hands exposed) in mid-morning or late afternoon, at least three times a week from April through October. If you go out when the sun's rays are stronger, say, at noon, be sure to use a sunscreen after the first few minutes of exposure. (You never need to burn to make adequate vitamin D.) Since sunscreens with a sun protection factor higher than 8 totally block the skin's ability to make vitamin D, coat yourself after you've received your dose of sun.

"If you don't want to bother with the sun and you can't or won't drink milk," says Dr. Holick, "you can take a multivitamin supplement containing 200 to 400 international units of vitamin D." But don't take more than 400 international units per day from a supplement, because high levels can be toxic.

Dr. Holick also advises elderly people to ask their physicians to have levels of the circulating form of vitamin D (25-hydroxy vitamin D) checked once or twice a year.

Strategy 3: Estrogen

We don't usually think of taking a drug as a preventive step, but estrogen replacement therapy (ERT) now appears to be the single most effective means for preventing bone loss and fractures in postmenopausal women. And in some circumstances, it can be a bone saver for younger women, too.

As its name implies, ERT replaces losses of natural

estrogen that occur with menopause or for other reasons. In ERT, you take small doses of estrogen in pill form or wear a self-adhesive patch that transmits it through your skin.

In general, whether you have bone loss or not, ERT is recommended if you experience early menopause (before the late forties), either naturally or because the ovaries have been surgically removed. But ERT is also in order if you've had a bone-mass measurement test showing significant losses.

In the fight against osteoporosis, the need for ERT—and its benefits—varies with age.

Young Adulthood to Middle Age ▶ If young or middle-aged women exercise excessively—to the point that they stop menstruating—they can be estrogen deficient and lose bone tissue. The problem occurs most often in distance runners. Women with eating disorders can have this problem, too. B. Lawrence Riggs, M.D., president of the National Osteoporosis Foundation and professor of medical research at Mayo Medical School, says that young women who fit either of these descriptions should have bone-mass measurement tests. (See "How Do You Know If You Have Osteoporosis?" on page 140.) If the test results are below normal, ERT is probably appropriate until a behavioral change can be made. (The problem is that compulsive exercisers and women with eating disorders often refuse ERT because it can cause some fluid weight gain.)

Around Menopause ▶ Women going through or just completing menopause can benefit most from ERT because this is the time when the most rapid bone loss occurs.

When started early, ERT can actually help women recoup lost bone. As for fractures, when started within a few years of the onset of menopause, women who take ERT have fewer broken bones than those who do not take it. ERT is most effective if started in early menopause and continued for at least ten years. Dr. Riggs advises that all women evaluate the pros and cons of ERT with their physicians around the time of menopause. Anyone who is concerned about osteoporosis and who would be willing to be on long-term ERT if test results were subnormal should have a bone-mass measurement test. If the test results show your bone mass is in the lower one-third of the normal range for your age, then you're a candidate for ERT. Women in the upper third are likely protected. Those in between should probably have a repeat bone test in two or three years to see if ERT would be appropriate.

Beyond Menopause ▶ Older women or women who have more advanced osteoporosis can probably benefit from ERT, too, although not as much as younger women. According to Robert Lindsay, M.D., professor of clinical medicine at the College of Physicians and Surgeons of Columbia University, benefits may result at any age up to around age 70. The major advantage is slowing of further bone loss.

Despite its bone-sparing benefits, only a small percentage of postmenopausal women are on long-term ERT for bone protection. Dr. Riggs says that most osteoporosis researchers would probably agree that more women should be.

So why are so few taking it? Partly because so many people aren't aware of its advantages; partly because it's not risk-free. Women taking estrogen all by itself have an increased risk of endometrial cancer. Risk increases from 1 case of cancer per 1,000 women to 4 per 1,000. To minimize this risk, another female hormone, progesterone, is usually prescribed along with estrogen. (Progesterone may not be necessary in women who have had a hysterectomy.)

It's also thought that ERT may increase risk of breast cancer. All women should have frequent manual breast exams and a mammogram both before starting ERT and every year thereafter. In general, women who've had breast cancer should not be started on ERT. Other con-

103

HOW DO YOU KNOW IF YOU HAVE OSTEOPOROSIS?

Ordinary x-rays, standard lab tests, or a physical exam can't reliably indicate if you have osteoporosis. Unfortunately, the first tip-off of osteoporosis often comes when someone fractures a bone. But it doesn't have to get that bad before the disease is detected. Now there are noninvasive ways to measure bone mass in different parts of the body in order to predict the likelihood of a fracture.

The fancy names of the only tests that can reliably measure bone mass and assess fracture risk are single-photon absorptiometry (SPA), dual-photon absorptiometry (DPA), quantitative computed tomography (QCT), and dual-energy x-ray absorptiometry (DEXA). All these tests take a more sensitive picture of bones than x-rays can. They use photons (units of magnetic energy), which are absorbed at a different rate by bone than by soft tissue and so reveal bone density on film.

The tests vary in the amount of radiation exposure. But all methods are considered safe, with radiation doses no higher than those of a full dental x-ray. Besides, bone-mass measurement tests are done infrequently.

ditions that may prohibit ERT include vaginal bleeding, active liver disease, severe, uncontrolled high blood pressure, and active thrombophlebitis and/or thromboembolus (both clotting disorders).

On the plus side, ERT can ease some menopause-related symptoms, including hot flashes, vaginal dryness, moodiness, insomnia, and excessive perspiration. ERT may protect against heart disease in older women, but progesterone may diminish the positive effects.

The most common indication for having a bone-mass measurement is in women who are estrogen deficient because of natural or artificial menopause (for example, when ovaries are removed). Other indicators include smoking, alcohol consumption of over two drinks a day, family history of the disease, being Caucasian and petite, and thyroid and cortisone therapy.

Osteoporosis researcher C. Conrad Johnston, M.D., of the University of Indiana School of Medicine, advises a bone-mass measurement test for any postmenopausal woman who would be willing to take estrogen-replacement therapy if the results were below normal.

Mass screening of all perimenopausal women isn't recommended, in part because insurance companies don't always reimburse for bone-mass measurements. But if you and your physician feel you're a candidate for screening, there seem to be no major differences in the four tests in their ability to predict fracture risk.

The decision to stop ERT should be based on the benefits and risks, which should be reviewed each year with your physician. It's imperative for women on ERT to keep their regular medical appointments so any side effects will be caught early.

Dr. Lindsay stresses that ERT cannot be considered in a vacuum. It's important to keep up your calcium intake at the same time. Continuing exercise is important, too.

Strategy 4: Exercise

Exercise seems to be good for your bones—old or young. "All you have to do is look at the forearm of a tennis player to see the effect of exercise—not only is the muscle overdeveloped, but the bone is larger, too," says Everett Smith, Ph.D., director of the Biogerontology Laboratory at the University of Wisconsin. "Bone is very much like muscle. If you exercise it, it gets bigger. If you stop, it atrophies." Exercise can also allow you to eat more without gaining weight, making it easier to get plenty of calcium.

Exercise's positive effects on bones can vary according to age.

Young Women ▶ Research indicates that women in their twenties who exercise have more bone than those who don't. Excessive, to-the-limit workouts at this age, though, can lower the body's production of estrogen, adversely affecting bone.

Middle-Aged Women ▶ We know now that regular exercise may slow bone loss in premenopausal and post-menopausal women. It can increase bone mass in some postmenopausal women. Dr. Smith published a study in which he and his colleagues looked at the effect of exercise on bone loss in a group of 35- to 65-year-old women. They compared 62 nonexercising women with 80 who did endurance dancing for 45 minutes a day, three times a week. (Endurance dancing is similar to low-impact aerobics, but you move the whole width and length of a gym, and it taxes many different parts of the body.) After four years, the exercisers had lost significantly less bone in their arms (the only bones the researchers measured) than did the nonexercisers. Whether they were premenopausal or postmenopausal, exercisers had lower bone loss rates.

Dr. Smith emphasizes that exercise will not replace ERT for women who need it, but exercise is important for all women, whether on ERT or not. Adequate exercise and calcium are both important for maintaining bone regardless of age or menopausal status.

Whatever your age, bone experts stress the importance of weight-bearing exercise for bones in the hip and spine. By weight bearing, they mean exercise that you do in an upright position—like walking, jogging, hiking, tennis, dancing, low-impact aerobics, stair climbing, and cross-country skiing.

Dr. Heaney maintains that you may get the most benefit for your bones by doing lots of different types of exercise. Dr. Smith agrees: "You should do a variety of weight-bearing exercises at least three or four days a week for 50 minutes."

An ideal program, in his opinion: Three days a week, do something aerobic, where you're moving in a variety of different directions—dancing, tennis, racquetball, or walking. Another two days, do exercise to strengthen your upper body—forearms, upper arms, chest, and shoulder area. For this, Dr. Smith advises weight training, elastic-tubing exercises, using a rowing machine, or using strength-training equipment. (Those who already have osteoporosis should consult their physician before starting any exercise program.) "Further research is needed to define the effects of strength training on bone mass," says Dr. Smith. "But we do know that it improves muscular strength, which can protect against falls."

If you're just starting to exercise, get your physician's okay first. Then proceed slowly, increasing your activity a little at a time.

Strategy 5: New Frontiers

Several compounds are currently under investigation—but not yet approved by the Food and Drug Administration (FDA)—for prevention and treatment of osteoporosis.

Diphosphonates ▶ These work by coating bone crystal, thereby preventing bone loss. Taken orally, they're used intermittently (taken perhaps 14 days in a row at the beginning of every three months). You may have heard about a study that showed dramatic results when a group of postmenopausal women with osteoporosis were treated with etidronate, a diphosphonate. Not only did women receiving etidronate for two years have significant increases in spinal bone mass, but the rate of new vertebral fractures was cut to half that of untreated women.

While etidronate is available for treating Paget's disease, it has not yet been approved by the FDA for use in osteoporosis. It appears similar to ERT in its effect on bone but without the hormonal side effects.

Calcitonin ▶ This is a hormone extracted from salmon (but naturally occurring in our body). When taken by injection (the usual approach) or by nasal spray (awaiting FDA approval), calcitonin can slow bone breakdown and relieve pain.

The hormone is especially useful for people who are at risk for osteoporosis but can't take ERT (perhaps because they've had breast cancer or they're male).

Fluoride ▶ This drug (in the form of sodium fluoride) is the stuff that makes kids' teeth strong. It may, in much higher doses, help people with established osteoporosis, because it can stimulate bone formation. But current data fail to show its benefit in preventing fractures, since the new bone produced may be of irregular structure and possibly of inferior strength.

For more information on osteoporosis, plus a booklet, send $2 to the National Osteoporosis Foundation, 2100 M Street NW, Suite 602, Dept. PM, Washington, DC 20037.

13 Nutrients on the Antiaging Frontier

Imagine old age without arthritis, cataracts, osteoporosis, and memory loss. Imagine being able to stave off cancer and heart disease indefinitely. You may not need to have a rich imagination to picture a healthy old age. You may be able to live it.

Welcome to nutrition's "brave new world." New research, much of it done at the U.S. Department of Agriculture's Human Nutrition Research Center on Aging (HNRC) at Tufts University in Boston, may yet make it possible to grow old gracefully, without growing chronically ill and infirm.

Through proper diet—with the right amounts and kinds of nutrients—we may be able to remain healthy throughout the life that medical research and technology is prolonging.

Following is an exclusive interview with Jeffrey Blumberg, Ph.D., associate director of HNRC. (HNRC recently celebrated its tenth anniversary as the only research center in the country whose sole purpose is to study the relationship between nutrition and the aging process.)

Q: Everybody's looking for an easy answer; how close are we to an antiaging supplement?

A: I wish I could say we're almost there, but I don't think we'll ever find a single magic bullet. Life is more complicated.

Currently, however, I must say vitamins E and B_6 are showing a lot of promise in our antiaging research. We have done some exciting studies with these two nutrients; it appears that they affect the health of the immune system. Generally, immunity declines somewhat as we get older, making us more susceptible to bacterial and viral infections, as well as certain diseases most common among the elderly, like cancer, arthritis, and heart disease.

Several studies have shown that certain nutrients, especially the so-called antioxidants (vitamins E and C and beta-carotene), may slow or prevent the decline in immunity. Our most striking work in this area was with vitamin E supplements in older people. We found that high doses markedly improved certain tests of immune function. For instance, when we did a skin patch test exposing the skin to certain toxins, the person should have reacted with a red swelling (caused when the immune system increases its output of white blood cells that surround and destroy the toxin). This would show that their immune system is responding and fighting the antigen. In older people, we found this response didn't occur because their immune system is less vigorous. However, after giving older people vitamin E supplements, their response to the skin patch test was like that of younger people.

More recently, we found that vitamin B_6 might play a role in the proper functioning of the immune system, too. Two other HNRC members, Robert Russell, M.D., professor of medicine at Tufts Medical School, and Simin Meydani, Ph.D., associate professor of nutrition at Tufts School of Nutrition, discovered that when healthy, elderly people had vitamin B_6 almost completely taken out of their diet, their immune response went down, as expected. What wasn't anticipated was the finding that the amount of vitamin B_6 needed to restore immune function was much higher than the current Recommended Dietary Allowance (RDA) of about 2 milligrams. And when the study participants were provided with higher than the RDA levels, their immune function was even better than it was before the study started! A word of caution, however: Vitamin B_6 can be toxic at 25 times the RDA.

Q: Are you suggesting that the RDA for certain vitamins might not be high enough to put the brakes on the illnesses that accompany aging?

A: I believe that, for some nutrients, the RDAs should probably be increased as we age; in other cases, however, the RDAs may need to be lowered for older adults since the need for certain nutrients seems to decrease as we age.

Keep in mind that the RDAs are nutritional guidelines designed to help prevent deficiency symptoms in the average healthy person. But there is a growing number of studies that suggest that the RDAs are not really appropriate or sensitive to the changing nutritional needs of aging adults. Nor are they focused on the most important public health objectives today—preventing chronic diseases like cancer and heart disease.

In most cases, the RDAs are extrapolations based on studies of younger people. If you look at the current RDAs you'll see that although there are special amounts for children and younger adults, there really aren't special amounts for people over age 51. But we're finding that the needs of younger adults are not the same as those of people in their sxities, seventies, and eighties.

Take the vitamin B_6 study we were just talking about as an example. While it was only a preliminary study, it does suggest the need for vitamin B_6 may increase with age, and even higher amounts of vitamin B_6 might prevent or delay age-related changes in the immune system. More research needs to be done, however, before we can make any specific recommendations. (Taking more than 50 milligrams a day of vitamin B_6 can be harmful.)

Q: You mentioned that certain nutrients, called antioxidants, have been shown to slow down the deterioration that accompanies aging. How do they work?

A: Nutrients such as vitamins E and C and beta-carotene may slow down or prevent damage from chemicals called free radicals. Free radicals occur naturally, for instance, when the fat and proteins you eat interact with the oxygen in your body to form toxic compounds. When there are too many free radicals, they can attack parts of your body's cells, like cell membranes, causing them to break down. There is a theory that aging is the result of accumulated damage from free radical reactions. Fortunately, Mother Nature has provided a natural way to cope with free radicals, in the form of these antioxidants. Antioxidants help inactivate free radicals and prevent them from attacking cells. Each one seems to work in a different way to counteract free radical damage, so they're all important.

Even if free radical reactions don't cause aging per se, a growing body of evidence suggests they are involved in immune function decline, as well as in causing common

111

∎

age-related diseases, including heart disease and cancer. Based on experimental studies, some researchers believe anti· ·idants may help prevent these ailments.

As a case in point, a Harvard Medical School study revealed that 333 men with heart disease who were given beta-carotene supplements for an average of six years had fewer heart attacks and heart-related deaths than did men not given the supplements. Again, the study is preliminary. We don't know whether beta-carotene plays a preventive role for people who don't have heart disease.

Q: Is there any way to get a jump on stalling the aging process, say, by increasing our intake of certain nutrients while in middle age?

A: My feeling is that if we can retard or reverse a phenomenon like the decline in immunity with nutritional intervention in older adults, then it's reasonable to speculate that we can slow age-related changes by having a relatively high intake of these nutrients in the middle years. Since research in this area is still in early stages, however, it will be years before we know whether certain vitamins—and what amounts—slow aging. We do know changes in the immune system—and in nutrient needs—are gradual. So I think it makes sense to pay special attention to your diet, increasing intake of nutritional foods, before you reach old age.

Q: With weight control a growing concern for many of us as we grow older, the question is: How do we eat more foods without consuming more calories?

A: The most obvious way is to focus on foods that contain the greatest concentration of nutrients with the least amount of calories and fat. Most fresh fruits and vegetables, whole grains, lean meats and fish, and low-fat or nonfat dairy products do that. (See "Youth-Full Foods" on page 114.) Don't waste your calories on sugary soft drinks, sweet confections, or alcohol—the so-called empty-calorie foods.

Exercise can also help. By virtue of the fact that you're burning off more calories, you can eat more food than someone who doesn't exercise. When you eat more food, you have a better chance of getting more vitamins and minerals. Exercise can also optimize the way the body handles certain nutrients. Calcium, for instance, seems to be incorporated into bone more efficiently if you exercise regularly.

Q: How do we ensure getting adequate amounts of vitamin E and other fat-soluble vitamins, which are found in polyunsaturated fats, if we eat a low-fat diet?

A: This is a major problem. Not only are many health-conscious people cutting back on fats of all types, but also the polyunsaturated fats that are on the market tend to have less vitamin E than they used to because of processing methods. In fact, a study published in the *Journal of the Canadian Dietetic Association* indicated that people who went from a diet containing more than 30 percent fat calories to one providing less fat experienced a drop in vitamin E intake that placed them well below RDA levels. Even RDA amounts may not be enough to optimize immune function as we grow older. This may be one case when supplementation may be in order. Many vitamin E researchers suggest supplements of 100 to 400 international units per day; however, there aren't enough studies yet to be more specific than that.

Q: You mentioned calcium. It's quite clear that having adequate dietary calcium when you're young helps protect against osteoporosis. But does it do any good to up calcium intake past middle age?

A: Yes. In fact, Bess Dawson-Hughes, M.D., and her colleagues in our Calcium and Bone Metabolism Laboratory published a study on calcium supplementation in postmenopausal women in the *New England Journal of Medicine*. They concluded that women who are six or more years past menopause, whose normal diet provides less than 400 milligrams of calcium, which is half the RDA (pretty common in this country), can significantly reduce bone loss if they increase their calcium intake to 800 milligrams a day. I think most postmeno-

YOUTH-FULL FOODS

Research on the aging process—like that coming out of the U. S. Department of Agriculture Human Nutrition Research Center on Aging at Tufts University—suggests that maximizing the nutritional quality of your diet may slow down or prevent age-related problems that many people think of as inevitable. The following are top food sources of key nutrients that have shown promise in antiaging research. (Since a number of these nutrients are destroyed by light and air, store foods in airtight containers and avoid light exposure. Also cook foods for as short a time and in as little water as possible.)

Vitamin E (RDA: 10 milligrams for men; 8 milligrams for women). Good sources: wheat germ, peanut butter, almonds, filbert nuts, sunflower seeds, shrimp, and vegetable oils. Green leafy vegetables also supply vitamin E.

Vitamin C (RDA: 60 milligrams for men and women). Good sources: citrus fruits and juices, strawberries, red and green peppers, broccoli, cantaloupe, and fortified juices. Also, potatoes (white and sweet), mangoes, tomatoes (and juice), watermelon, honeydew, brussels sprouts, snow peas, and cauliflower.

pausal women need more. Although 800 milligrams may slow down bone loss, the body is still losing calcium at this level; 1,200 to 1,500 milligrams a day has been recommended for postmenopausal women who are not on estrogen (estrogen helps maintain bone density); 1,000 milligrams if you're on estrogen or you've not yet entered menopause.

114

Q: Also, if you're getting your calcium from supplements rather than foods, aren't you missing out on

Beta-carotene (RDA: none). Good sources: carrots, winter squash, pumpkin, sweet potatoes, dark green vegetables (like spinach, kale, and broccoli), apricots, cantaloupe, mangoes, and peaches.

Vitamin B$_6$ (RDA: 2 milligrams for men; 1.6 milligrams for women). Good sources: chicken, fish, lean pork, and eggs. Also whole grain rice, soybeans, oats, whole wheat products, peanuts, bananas, plantains, and walnuts.

Vitamin B$_{12}$ (RDA: 2 micrograms for men and women). Good sources: lean meats and fish. Also milk products and eggs.

Folate (RDA: 200 micrograms for men; 180 micrograms for women). Good sources: legumes, such as lentils, kidney beans, and black-eyed peas, citrus fruits, whole grain products, and vegetables, particularly spinach.

Calcium (RDA: 800 milligrams for men and women; 1,200 milligrams for pregnant and lactating women). Good sources: dairy products, broccoli, kale, collards, and sardines.

Note that fortified cereals may provide fair amounts of some or all of these nutrients. Check the labels, since products vary.

vitamin D, which is added to milk and so important in helping your body use the calcium?

A. You may be. Since vitamin D is needed to absorb and metabolize calcium in the body, it's another important nutrient for keeping bones "young" and strong. But several factors get in the way of vitamin D metabolism as we grow older. Not only does the body become less efficient at converting vitamin D from foods and supplements to a usable form, but the skin is less efficient at making the vitamin when it's exposed to the sun. In addition, recent studies by Dr. Dawson-Hughes and Elizabeth Krall, Ph.D., here at Tufts show that older women who consume less than 200 international units of vitamin D a day—which is the current RDA—have an increase in parathyroid hormone in the wintertime. Now, parathyroid hormone breaks down bone, so this study suggests that in the winter you're breaking down bone at a greater rate.

On the other hand, women who consumed more than 200 international units of vitamin D a day did not have this seasonal increase in parathyroid hormone. This is an important finding because it suggests that the seasonal breakdown in bone can be prevented with adequate vitamin D—but an absolute minimum is 200 international units. If we take into account individual variation in needs, I think a more appropriate level is about 400 international units, which would satisfy the requirements of those with higher needs while still maintaining a safe level. You'll find that amount in many supplements. And every cup of milk has 100 international units of vitamin D. (Remember that too much vitamin D can be harmful.)

Q: There's been a lot of talk lately that being underweight may actually prolong your life. But aren't very thin people at risk for osteoporosis?

A: It's true that for some reason very thin individuals are at higher risk for osteoporosis. Remember, though, that osteoporosis is related to a combination of risk factors ranging from low calcium intake to low estrogen levels, as well as inactivity. But as far as longevity is concerned, I don't think that there's much sound evidence that being underweight prolongs human life. Yes, numerous studies in rats and mice show that animals fed diets that are deficient in calories but adequate in protein, vitamins, and minerals tend to live longer than animals fed normal diets. The problem is that these studies have only been done in animals that have very short life spans, and the findings may or may not apply to humans. We'll have a better answer years from now when ongoing studies in monkeys (which have much longer life spans and are biologically more like people) are completed by the National Institute on Aging (NIA).

Q: So cutting back on calories isn't a good idea if you're trying to stay younger longer.

A: I don't recommend caloric restriction, because it's very experimental. Animals in caloric restriction studies are "undernourished but not malnourished." They're on carefully planned diets that assure the animals are getting the right nutrients. People who try this on their own could easily become malnourished. All along we've been talking about how important it is to have a nutrient-rich diet if you want to slow aging. That becomes much tougher if you cut way back on calories.

Q: Do you mean it's okay to get fat as you grow older?

A: We're not talking about becoming obese or about people who were already overweight. This just suggests that maybe it's good to have a little fat reserve when you're older so that if you do develop some sort of disease, you've got something to draw upon. Being a little heavier may also act as a hedge against the natural decline in appetite that tends to occur as we age. I'd say that if you were not overweight when you were younger, then you certainly shouldn't panic if you weigh up to about 5 percent more than your youthful weight during middle age.

Q: What about where people gain weight? Isn't that important? We've heard a lot recently about the "apple" and "pear" shapes and their relation to disease.

A: There's no question that people who tend to gain weight around the middle—our so-called apple-shaped people—are at higher risk for problems like heart disease, hypertension, and diabetes than are pear-shaped individuals who pack the extra weight on their hips and buttocks. A healthy weight for "apples" is probably less than that for "pears." Also, if you have a medical problem

117

that's aggravated by weight, such as hypertension, you may benefit from being on the slim side.

Remember, no matter what you weigh, your goal should be to keep up your lean body or muscle tissue by exercising. Since muscle tissue burns fat but fat tissue doesn't, that should help boost your calorie requirement. Thus, if you're exercising you can afford more calories.

Q: Are you saying that if we're nutritionally fit, we're more likely to maintain a leaner, more muscular physique as we age?

A: We have supporting evidence from our exercise physiology laboratory, where William Evans, Ph.D., and his co-workers have done a series of studies to examine the impact of fairly intensive exercise training—involving a combination of activities like bicycling, walking, and weight lifting—on people of various ages. Not surprisingly, people who exercised more were the most physically fit—whether they were young or as old as 90. What came as a surprise was the finding that the extent to which exercise helped a person maintain muscle mass seemed to depend on how "nutritionally fit" he or she was.

In one study, Dr. Evans put people on an exercise program and gave them a liquid supplement containing a variety of vitamins and minerals, as well as protein. He found that this regimen seemed to increase both muscle mass and strength in older people, but made no difference in young adults. Since the supplement contained many different nutrients, we don't know which one or ones might have been responsible for the improvement. But the fact that the participants were all eating pretty well-balanced diets indicates that getting extra amounts of one or more nutrients might optimize the effect of exercise in middle-aged and older adults.

Q: Is there anything we can do to keep our brain as healthy as our aging body? Many people fear the loss of mental acuity more than they fear some of the killer diseases.

A: There's some exciting new research going on now aimed at keeping the brain young. For a long time we've known that people who are seriously deficient in B vitamins start to develop mental or cognitive troubles, as well as other problems, such as anemia. But we now have sophisticated tests that tell us when people are just borderline deficient—when they show no outward or obvious signs of deficiency—in vitamins B_6, B_{12}, and folate. When someone is borderline deficient in any of these nutrients, levels of an amino acid called homocysteine become elevated. There's evidence that a small but significant number of elderly people have elevated homocysteine levels that return to normal when the mild deficiencies are corrected with B-vitamin supplements. Not only that, but preliminary studies suggest some people show improvement in memory and learning ability after B supplementation.

Q: So what does this mean for younger people who want to stay sharp to a ripe old age?

A: Based on the limited evidence we have, I'd say that changes in cognitive function are gradual. So you want to make sure that your diet is rich in these three nutrients—vitamins B_6, B_{12}, and folate—because they seem to be particularly vulnerable to the aging process. I don't mean to imply, however, that taking B vitamins will prevent or reverse all cognitive changes related to aging.

Q: Speaking of keeping sharp, what about the eyes? Is there any dietary way to preserve your vision as you grow older?

A: Most people don't realize that cataracts afflict virtually everyone who lives long enough. The process, which results in loss of transparency of the lens of the eye and eventual loss of vision, usually starts around age 60. Cataracts can be easily corrected with surgery, but who wants to go through the trouble and expense if you can avoid it? Since we now know that cataracts develop because of free radical damage to the lens—for example, as a result of exposure to ultraviolet light from the sun— it makes sense that antioxidants would play a protective role. Indeed, studies of older people by Paul Jacques, D.Sc., assistant professor of nutrition at Harvard University, showed that those with higher blood and dietary levels of vitamins E and C and beta-carotene had the lowest incidence of cataracts. Now I want to stress that this refers to a reduction in risk—some people who had high antioxidant levels also had cataracts. It may be that these people had more exposure to UV light when they were younger.

Q: So what's the bottom line for people who want to do everything in their power to put the brakes on aging through nutrition?

A: In essence, eating a superhigh-quality diet is crucial if you want to do all you can to stay young longer. It's especially important to key in on good food sources of vitamins E and C and beta-carotene. (See "Youth-Full

---

THE BEST ANTIAGING DIET KNOWN

Following these guidelines may help slow some of the effects of aging.

● Decrease fat to less than 30 percent of your overall calorie intake.

● Increase fiber to between 20 and 35 grams a day.

● Eat foods rich in the antioxidants—vitamins E and C and beta-carotene.

● Consume low-fat foods high in calcium.

● Take a multivitamin/mineral supplement to ensure you're getting at least the RDAs.

Foods.") It's interesting that it keeps coming back to these antioxidants—whether we're talking about immune function, cardiovascular disease, or cataracts. I'd work on eating good sources of B vitamins and folate as well. In addition, I'd go so far as to advise people who want to take steps to slow down the aging process to take a daily multivitamin/mineral supplement. Research so far suggests that if you're an older adult, you should take a multivitamin/mineral supplement formulated at one to two times the RDA levels, plus eat a diverse diet low in fat and high in fiber. The idea behind this is that then you can die "young"—as late as possible.

Sail Smoothly through Midlife 14

For many of us, the big four-oh marks the beginning of the big squeeze. Sandwiched as we are between growing children and aging parents—and feeling the pinch of mortality and reality—the pressure builds. Midlife crisis in the making? Not necessarily. Research shows—and several psychologists agree—that for those people who accept change as a challenge, the decade of the forties can be a period of accelerated growth, renewal, and fulfillment.

This, of course, stands in sharp contrast to the stereotypical view of midlife as a time of inescapable turmoil—when all hell breaks loose. But the new positive image of middle age is gaining ground—and not just among psychologists. When the American Board of Family Practice (ABFP) recently surveyed 1,200 Americans on their perspectives on middle age, they found overwhelmingly high expectations. More than 80 percent viewed middle age as a period of positive growth. They commonly described it as a time of caring and compassion and of deepening relationships between family and friends. What's more, there's a perception that midlifers have certain inherent advantages over their twenty- and thirtysomething siblings. They've got the wisdom that comes from experience, the greater financial security of an established career, and in many cases, the freedom to come and go without booking a babysitter. All of this, the surveyed people said, adds up to a greater sense of control.

Perception vs. Reality

"If you think you are getting happier as you get older, the research says you are right," says Margaret Gatz, Ph.D., a University of Southern California psychologist.

Dr. Gatz has studied levels of depression in four age groups (40 and under, 40 to 54, 55 to 69, and 70 and up) and found that those in the 40 to 54 age bracket are the second least likely to be depressed. The least likely to be depressed are those in the 55 to 69 age group.

"All of this makes tremendous sense," she explains. "In the midlife you are getting good at handling difficult situations that used to really throw you when you were younger." An added benefit of the middle years is a growing sense of identity. "Somewhere in the middle, you are getting hold of who you are—finally."

That's not to say we can expect to fly through our forties without any turbulence. Midlife is a transitional time, comparable in many ways to adolescence. Short of having bad skin, a person in "middlescence" can greatly resemble an adolescent who is confronted with sweeping change: physically, emotionally, psychologically, and socially.

"Like adolescents, 'middlescents' are drawn by change to explore the world within their internal world," says Nolan Brohaugh, a senior associate at the William Menninger Center for Applied Behavioral Sciences. Invariably, change triggers twinges of uncertainty and apprehension.

You might call these twinges midlife growing pains. Everyone feels them, but the question is, to what degree?

For some they may be incapacitating. For others they serve as healthy reminders that they are in a growth spurt.

Change as Opportunity

"It's interesting to note that, in Chinese, the word *crisis* is made up of two characters: one represents danger, the other opportunity," says Boston psychologist Joan Borysenko, Ph.D. "There will always be people who are devastated by change. But, more and more, we're finding people who view change as an opportunity rather than a threat."

Mark Gerzon, author of *The Midlife Quest,* agrees. "We turn midlife into a midlife crisis by pretending that everything is supposed to stay the same. But it isn't," he writes. "Based on my own experiences, the lives of others, and a review of fiction and scholarship about midlife, I am convinced that the second half of human life is a profound opportunity for transformation. It is a chance to live by new rules and to catch a second, and deeper, wind."

Dr. Borysenko says her own midlife transformation began as a head-on collision—literally. Driving home late one night, after another work-filled day, she fell asleep at the wheel and hit a car coming from the opposite direction.

Fortunately, the driver of the other car was not seriously injured. But while Dr. Borysenko lay recuperating in the hospital, her doctor suggested that her accident was a metaphor for life in the fast lane. She decided, then, that it was time to reorder her priorities.

"I realized how precious my family and friends were and how little time I had had for them," she recalls. At the time, Dr. Borysenko worked with renowned stress expert Herbert Benson, M.D., at the Mind/Body Clinic at the New England Deaconess Hospital. But ironically, she admits, "I was working too hard."

So she made some changes. She left the Mind/Body Clinic and formed a consulting business, which offers stress-reduction workshops. "Today I have a more rea-

123
∎

sonable schedule," she notes. "Also, as a result of my midlife crisis, I started to appreciate myself more. The experience made me reconsider all the ways I thought I was not good enough.

"I began to recognize the value of who I am as a human being, not just for what I do." Now, at 44, she concludes, "I'm much gentler with myself."

"Midlife is a period in which behavior comes into line with values," says Brohaugh.

"Many people begin to reassess their career goals in terms of satisfying their human rather than economic needs," says Neil Fiore, Ph.D., a Berkeley, California, psychologist and author of *The Now Habit: Overcoming Procrastination and Enjoying Guilt-Free Play.*

Typically, people decide at an early age what they are going to specialize in. After ten years or so they may feel bored or burned out.

They realize that job satisfaction has to do with the quality of their life, not just the power to buy consumer goods.

"And fortunately, with our improved health habits and increased life span, people are less afraid of making a change," says Dr. Fiore. Sometimes, too, it doesn't take a major change to bring about a better balance; small changes can make big differences. Maybe at age 40, Brohaugh points out, you realize that you aren't going to be the company president. Rather than stew over what could have been, consider what you've got. Then explore ways to use those skills and experiences to enhance your self-worth. Teach a course. Or think in even broader terms; maybe you've got what it takes to coach a Little League team. "This is a wonderful time to become a mentor," Brohaugh says.

The Intimacy/Industry Balance

In midlife, men and women often find themselves reevaluating (and struggling with) what Brohaugh calls the demands of intimacy and industry. "In their twenties and thirties, men are typically very interested in the industry part—in career, getting ahead, establishing financial support for their families," he says.

"And the intimacy side—closeness with wife (or husband) and children, nurturing the family, getting emotional gratification from close ties—gets deemphasized.

"Many women at the same age, though, balance intimacy and industry very differently. They spend most of their energy and time nurturing, loving, connecting with the ones they care about. And career, professional development, and the corporate ladder get ignored. Although for many women this pattern is beginning to change now.

"But in the forties, a switch begins. Men start to think, 'What really matters is not the job, the big bucks, but relationships, the family. When the chips are down, that's what really counts.' And women begin to think, especially if the kids have left home, 'I've put my career on hold for too long. I want to get my career started.' "

Being aware that this switch can happen puts you ahead of the game, Brohaugh says. You can then anticipate it, understand it more clearly, and maybe deal better with the transitions as they happen.

And the trick to dealing with them is to not let the intimacy/industry balancing act get out of balance.

"People in a relationship who let their own personal balancing of the two demands get lopsided are putting a strain on themselves and the relationship," Brohaugh says. "An arrangement in which the man is at one end of the scale and the woman is at another doesn't leave the couple with much common ground. So in the forties, when couples start to make the intimacy/industry switch, they need to avoid the extremes.

"In a healthy relationship, the man and woman typically take turns focusing on one aspect or the other. A man can be dependent on his wife, and then the next week he steps in and nurtures her."

The Power of Planning

125

Perhaps it is all of the midlife demands—community, family, the freedom of the empty nest, the challenge of breaking out of a rut, and even the never-ending battle of the bulge—that give so many people the chance to plan their midlife transition.

"To be forewarned is to be forearmed," says Don R. Powell, Ph.D., president of the American Institute for Preventive Medicine. "I think it is a good plan to know what is up the road. People in midlife have the base of wisdom with which to plan their lives. In our stress-management seminars we teach people goal setting, where they decide what goals they want to accomplish and over what period of time. Then we help people break down these goals into subgoals, which are essentially the behaviors they need to reach their big goals. Whether it is pursuing a new career or taking up a new hobby, it helps people feel in control."

A planned midlife transition is exactly what Dr. Fiore accomplished almost ten years ago. He was 38 then and a psychologist at the counseling center at the University of California, Berkeley. Having accomplished many of his professional goals, including publishing in the prestigious *New England Journal of Medicine,* Dr. Fiore planned a transition that would reduce counseling time 10 percent a year while he built up a private practice and speaking career. After five years, he had reduced his counseling time 50 percent. Today, he can happily say the planning paid off.

"I had a smooth and controlled transition and was able to ride through it because I planned it," he says. "Instead of it being a period of crisis, it turned into one of the best periods of my life."

Recognizing you may be headed for a crisis is the first step to smoothing out the bumps of midlife, says Dr. Borysenko. After all, you can't alter the course of change. But you can strengthen your stress-coping skills, So instead of feeling crushed by events, you can rise to the occasion. The following suggestions are designed to do just that: to help you create balance and harmony in your life and develop that all-important sense of control.

126

■ **Take a Moment to Become Mindful** ▶ What's more stressful than rationalizing with a teen? Or caring for an elderly parent? Or communicating with a difficult boss?

It's coping with all of these things; that's the forties for you. No wonder midlifers complain that life's out of control.

"Pretty soon you're overwhelmed. Then you ask, 'How can I begin to get a little peace of mind?'" says Jon Kabat–Zinn, Ph.D., director of the stress-reduction and relaxation program at the University of Massachusetts. "The only place to start is in a moment. That's what meditation is all about; it's being present in the moment—in other words, mindfulness.

"To help anchor you in the moment, just close your eyes and focus on your breathing," he explains. "Don't try to manipulate it, just observe it for a moment. Ride the waves of your breathing. If your mind starts to wander, gently bring it back to the breath and don't judge it.

"You don't have to stay with it for very long to eventually feel the effect. Try it for just 10 seconds or 30 seconds. Repeat it every hour or so. You can do it anywhere. Funny as it sounds, this is an incredibly powerful meditation technique," Dr. Kabat–Zinn maintains. "It helps you develop two things: concentration, or calmness, and mindfulness. As you notice your thoughts coming and going, you observe the actual play of the mind and the fact that it's constantly changing. That gives you a certain flexibility to respond to stressful events instead of reacting to them, which is our usual, automatic and mindless mode of operation."

Relish Life's Simple Pleasures ▶ Take the time to listen to the wind. Smell the lilacs. Savor a peach. "It's possible for people to get up and shuffle off to work barely noticing the nature around them. To spend all day indoors and never see the sun rise or set. To seldom be touched. To wolf down food and barely taste or enjoy it," says 41-year-old David Sobel, M.D., coauthor of the book *Healthy Pleasures*. "This deprivation is at a cost to one's well-being."

How does he manage stress? "I don't worry much about managing it," he says. "I simply try to fill my life with activities I find personally pleasurable, things that help rejuvenate me."

Dr. Borysenko takes a similar approach. "I'll go out for a walk with my husband and our dog, not only for exercise but because it's beautiful outside in nature and it's fun to watch the dog run through the woods."

Make Time to Play ▶ Unfortunately, once we pass childhood, play is no longer appreciated on its own merits; it's considered a means to an end. "We play golf for contacts and bowl for charity. How often do we play for the love of it?" Pennsylvania State University leisure expert Geoffrey Godbey, Ph.D., asks.

"A person in midlife transition can be addicted to work and feel guilty about playing," says Dr. Fiore. "If he isn't producing, he feels he is doing nothing. In fact, studies have shown that peak performers take more than the average number of holidays—at least six weeks a year."

The devotion to play is all-important, especially to people who find themselves in a deep midlife rut. In the ABFP report, for example, over 40 percent of men and women polled expect to take up active sports like tennis and skiing. They're the kinds of activities that other research says contribute to a person's psychological "stress resistance."

"I used to play with my son and think about all the work I should be doing instead," says Dr. Sobel. "Now I understand that playing with him is one of the most productive things that I can possibly do." If you're a little rusty and don't know where to begin, 47-year-old Dr. Godbey makes a few suggestions: "Hang around doggies and kids; they know how to play," he says. "When a dog puts its head down and cocks it to one side, lowers its front paws, and looks at you, he's ready to roll."

Of course, any activity that you enjoy—whether gardening, painting, or having picnics in the park—is a worthwhile pursuit.

If you're having trouble with this, Dr. Fiore suggests you keep an "unschedule." That is, a calendar on which you schedule only play—walks in the park, tennis games, even time to goof off. Then fill your work schedule in around the good times.

Build Intimate Bonds ▶ Learn to open up to others, to share your deepest feelings, and to instill in others the trust to do the same. Psychologists tell us that intimacy is not only an immediate stress reducer, it provides the kind of loving, nonjudgmental support that helps us develop confidence to deal with whatever life sends our way.

Give ▶ It's been said that the twenties are a time when we focus on our marriage; the thirties a time to focus on career; and the forties, "a time to give something back," says Brohaugh. "Try it. You'll find that altruism is its own reward."

Looking Fabulous at 40-Plus   15

No one can turn back the years—then again, you don't have to. Today you can look better in your forties than you've ever looked. Science understands more about the factors that age skin and can offer more help and preventive measures than ever before. It's not too late to undo at least some of the damage that may have been done in the past and, more important, head off some of the formerly inevitable signs of aging. Among the factors that contribute to your appearance, there's one you don't have power over—genetics. But there are plenty of others you do control.

The Antagonists

"The number-one contributor to how old your skin looks is ultraviolet sun damage," says Ronald Sherman,

M.D., senior clinical instructor in dermatology at Mount Sinai Medical Center in New York City. "It destroys the ability of your skin to renew itself at peak capacity." Mostly because of sun damage, in your forties your smile and frown lines may deepen, crow's-feet may appear, and your skin may start to get blotchy.

The severity of your skin's reaction to sun damage is inherited. (If your parents showed the signs of sun damage in their forties, you should be doubly cautious of the sun yourself.) But you determine how much sun exposure you get.

Another factor is nutrition. The average American's diet contains more than adequate nutrition for the development of good hair, skin, and nails. However, if you respond to life stresses by overeating, skipping meals, or not eating properly, you can sabotage this natural advantage.

Lack of activity can also sabotage your efforts to look younger. Exercise is a vital component of beauty because it helps nourish your skin from the inside. "Regular exercise enhances the entire cardiovascular system, which, in turn, aids blood flow to the skin," says Rodney Basler, M.D., assistant professor of internal medicine, Division of Dermatology, University of Nebraska Medical Center. "This increases your skin's supply of nutrients and oxygen. Along with the increased blood flow it helps give your skin the glow and vitality we associate with an athlete."

Exercise greatly determines how you carry yourself. It promotes the strength and suppleness necessary for youthful-looking posture. If you were an actress playing the role of a 20-year-old, you'd straighten your back, throw back your shoulders, and tip up your chin.

Well, why should this be a role? Exercise can help make this the real you. And if you move like a 20-year-old, that's the impression you'll leave with people.

To complement this look of vitality, well-groomed skin, hair, and nails are essential. Don't underestimate the effects of such surface care. The most glowing skin looks unhealthy with the wrong makeup; the most glorious hair ages you if the style is unbecoming.

Another essential to looking your best that's frequently overlooked is attitude. "I see many potentially beautiful 30-, 40-, or 50-year-old women who've obviously spent considerable time and money on their appearance," says 40-year-old Trish McEvoy, of Dr. Ronald Sherman and Trish McEvoy Skin Care Center in New York City, who is a walking advertisement for what the forties can be.

"But their facial expressions—tension, anger—are very aging. For me, being 40 is as if I'm growing into my own skin. I've come to understand that you have to work for tomorrow but live in and appreciate what you have today."

The 40-Plus "Antiaging" Plan

So there are plenty of areas where you can do a lot of good. From top dermatologists and beauty experts come these practical strategies for exploiting every one of them for great looks at 40-plus.

Never Go into the Light of Day without Sun Protection ▶ This is the single most important thing you can do for your skin. If your moisturizer doesn't contain a sunscreen, apply one 20 minutes before you put on your makeup.

The thin, delicate skin around your eyes is usually the first place to show wrinkling caused by ultraviolet damage. Help prevent this by wearing UV-screening sunglasses year-round. Glasses shield the eye area and help keep you from the squinting that deepens crow's-feet.

Recalibrate Your Moisturizing System ▶ The forties are a time when people find that products and techniques that worked for years may not be appropriate any longer. As time passes, the sebaceous glands in the skin

131
■

that resupply oil slow down production. It's up to you to replace that moisture with a richer product formulated to your skin's new requirements.

For optimum effect, moisturizer is best applied after you've washed, while your skin is still damp, to seal the precious water next to your skin. Hands, feet, and neck can really give away your age. Be sure to use moisturizers and sunscreen in these areas.

Don't Use High-Alcohol Astringents and Skin Scrubs ▶ Skin that's fortysomething requires a gentler approach than it did in previous decades. Products containing alcohol can be drying.

Try 40-Plus Hair Care and Cut ▶ Nick Berardi, a senior hairstylist for Vidal Sassoon, offers these guidelines.

■ Always use a conditioner. In your forties, dry hair often becomes a problem as your scalp becomes drier and there are more coarse gray hairs.

■ Go with color or perm—not both. Each process tends to be drying, and together they can throw your hair into a vicious circle that leaves it dull and overdried.

■ Keep hair length above the shoulders. "This is a personal preference," says Berardi. "But I feel it shouldn't be longer because it looks not youthful but young looking." Also, hair that's gray often is wiry and responds much better to a shorter style.

■ If you want to color gray hair, instead of just covering it with a single color, try a process called tricolor lowlighting. "This uses your gray hair as one color," explains Barardi, "then weaves two other colors in that blend with your natural shade to give a warm, textured effect."

Use Subtle Makeup for Smashing Results ▶ A common mistake is that, as women feel that they have more to hide, they apply more foundation. This only leads to makeup collecting in the creases. A lightweight foundation looks good if you're 16 or 60. For a sheer application, apply your foundation with a sponge.

Use colors with a matte finish. Avoid frosted eye and lip colors. The frost settles in the fine lines and makes them more noticeable.

To hide dark blotches and forestall further darkening, use concealer with sunscreen or sunblock.

The
Healing
Power
of Herbs

Cream of the Herbal Crop

By Varro E. Tyler, Ph.D.

Mix in quinine's tartness, cascara's purgative power, asafetida for that medicinal smell, and a dollop of senna—another laxative—just for good measure. That's the formula for Long's Cold Capsules and my introduction to herbal remedies in T. J. Long's Pharmacy. I spent my teen summers working there in Nebraska City, Nebraska. Did T. J. Long's remedy work? I can't say for sure, but T.J. could rest assured that at least his customers knew something was happening. Today, as a specialist in natural remedies, I advise against home-brewed herbal laxatives. That's one situation where I think it's safer to trust the precisely measured dose of commercial preparations (many of which do contain herbal products).

But there's no question about it—science is getting a better handle on which herbs work and are not harmful. So the opportunity for safe, sane, and effective use of herbal remedies has increased.

The trick in using herbal remedies is to use common sense. This means, first of all, realizing that some herbs—even a few with sterling reputations in folklore—are dangerous. So you should try only those herbals that, for good scientific reasons, are deemed safe . . . like the herbs I catalog in this article. If you have a serious illness or severe symptoms, get medical advice or treatment first, before trying any herbal.

By the way, I never recommend herbals for infants and children. You can't predict an herb's effect on a tiny body with an immature metabolism. And in some cases herbs that are safe for adults can be outright harmful to kids. Peppermint's menthol, for instance, can make babies choke.

Another fact you have to keep in mind is that herbs lack standardization. This means you could buy the same herb from ten different sources and get something completely different every time. In fact, an analysis reported in *Lancet* a few years back found some commercial feverfew products contained no feverfew at all. In most cases, your best bet is to grow your own herb plants in your garden or on your windowsill. For most of the seven herbs listed here, I'm going to give you some tips on how to do just that. If you do try a commercial product and it doesn't work within a reasonable time, you may have to switch to another brand.

I'm going to tell you what the scientific facts are behind these herbs, how to use them and how not to. I consider these specimens of "natural medicine" safe (when used properly) and your best bets for herbal healing.

Aloe

Slippery aloe gel soothes the pain of almost any minor burn, scrape, or skin irritation. Studies also show it sharpens skin's healing skills. Aloe has its limits, though. Don't try it on burns that penetrate below the skin surface or on ulcers larger than dime-size. In a remarkable study, aloe aided 18 people who'd had facial dermabrasion (sanding away scars). Researchers applied the usual wound dressing on one side of each face, the same dressing soaked in aloe gel on the other. Aloe's advantages: less swelling after two days, less crusting by day four, and 90 percent skin regrowth by day six, compared to only 40 to 50 percent on the aloe-free side. And aloe appeared to reduce throbbing, although it stung when applied. The researchers calculate that aloe speeded up overall wound healing time by three days.

While many people swear by aloe vera juice for various ailments, long-term internal use is not a good idea. Aloe contains chemicals called anthraquinones—potent stimulants of the colon. Prolonged use can lead to "lazy bowel syndrome," whereby the bowel relies on chemical stimulation to function normally.

Healing Techniques ▶ Cut a fleshy aloe plant leaf and slice it open lengthwise. Squeeze out enough of the clear gel to seal your wound. (Squiggles of yellow latex mean you're squeezing too hard. The latex should not be used.) Aloe works best in the open air, so leave your injury uncovered. Processed aloe gel may not give the same results as the freshly squeezed gel, so use fresh when possible.

Growing Tips ▶ Where winter temperatures dip below 41°F, grow warm-blooded aloe indoors on a sun-filled, south-facing windowsill. A vacation outdoors each summer should boost your aloe's growth.

Chamomile

The grande dame of herbal remedies, chamomile cradles potent volatile oils in its white-flowered crown. These oils seem to act two different ways: First, chamomile helps to ease violent smooth-muscle contractions, thereby halting stomach and menstrual cramps. Second, by exerting a soothing effect, as well as an analgesic action, on inflamed tissues, chamomile (when applied topically) may cool canker sores and mild skin irritations like dishpan hands.

One caution: Chamomile, like ragweed, is a member of the Daisy family, which you may be allergic to. So the prudent advice is, if you're allergic to ragweed, avoid chamomile. And even if you've never had a reaction to ragweed, any symptoms of hives, hay fever, or asthma mean that you should skip this remedy.

Healing Techniques ▶ For stomach or menstrual cramps, sip a very strong tea of 1 to 2 teaspoons of pulverized dried flower heads per cup of hot water, steeped for 10 to 15 minutes. This tea may be drunk three to four times a day. Swish the same brew in your mouth for 3 minutes to ease a canker sore. Mound moistened flower heads directly onto irritated skin.

Growing Tips ▶ I recommend planting annual chamomile seeds in the fall to get a head start on the next growing season. Plant in a sunny spot outdoors. Preserve dried flowers in an airtight container.

Cranberries

Cranberries are believed by many to help alleviate urinary tract infections (UTIs). There's no scientific proof of that yet (research is pending), but I believe that this remedy can't hurt and might help.

The common folk wisdom that acidic cranberry juice turns urine into a toxic bath for infectious bacteria, though, turns out to be wrong. Research suggests that cranberries actually prevent bacteria from anchoring on to bladder walls. So invaders can be swept away with each wave of urine.

Healing Techniques ▶ To possibly prevent UTIs, I recommend drinking 3 ounces of cranberry juice cocktail daily. If you should develop a UTI, drink 12 to 32 ounces of cocktail a day. Cranberry powder capsules lack the sugar that's added to sweeten the cocktail (a special advantage for diabetics). Six capsules equal 3 ounces of cranberry cocktail.

Feverfew

Feverfew may offer an herbal way to break the chains of migraine pain. A number of preliminary studies done in England suggest that feverfew may rein in both the frequency and severity of migraines, possibly by stemming the action of serotonin. Serotonin is the blood chemical most experts blame for kicking off migraine attacks. This research isn't proof, but I think it's at least strong enough for migraineurs to give feverfew a try, especially if they can't get relief otherwise.

For feverfew to work as a migraine exterminator, you have to chew on a few leaves every day. During the winter, or if chewing fresh leaves irritates your mouth, switch to the freeze-dried herb in capsule or tablet form. (Heat-dried feverfew is ineffective.) Feverfew is another branch of the Daisy family tree, so those with ragweed allergies should avoid it.

Healing Techniques ▶ Pick two or three small feverfew leaves each day (about 75 to 100 milligrams). Chew the leaves before swallowing them.

Growing Tips ▶ Ordinary, well-drained soil and full sunshine suit feverfew. Space plants 9 to 12 inches apart or sow seeds directly into the ground in early spring or fall.

Garlic

I think garlic has the biggest potential for healing of any of the herbs I selected for this list. In human studies, garlic seems to lower elevated cholesterol levels. Because garlic acts as a blood thinner, it may help protect against clogged arteries. Garlic also seems to act like a mild antibiotic and a digestive aid. There's even a whiff of evidence that garlic gourmands get less stomach and colorectal cancer. Garlic's only offense is imparting an odor problem that mouthwashes can't dent. Even encapsulated garlic doesn't help, because when the volatile oils are released in your stomach, they find their way to your pores, so you smell bad anyway.

Because garlic is an effective blood thinner, if you

GROW YOUR OWN

Shop nurseries in your own area for locally grown herbs starting in April. Or you can order plants from a mail-order nursery. One nursery that ships herbs is Well-Sweep Herb Farm, 317 Mount Bethel Road, Port Murray, NJ 07865. Send $2 for their catalog.

take daily aspirin or other blood-thinning drugs, or if you have a blood disorder, you should not use garlic supplements.

Healing Techniques ▶ I recommend eating real garlic. Eat it minced into a salad, in pasta sauce, or on garlic bread.

Growing Tips ▶ Plant garlic in early spring to harvest the following fall. Set cloves 2 inches deep and 6 inches apart in rich and dry soil. Full sun plumps up the thickest garlic bulbs.

Ginger

Ginger can be a lifesaver when you're riding waves of motion sickness. Nausea arises when your brain ex-

GINSENG'S ALLURE

Its reputation as an overall body invigorator and sex-stimulating elixir makes ginseng the most popular herb in this country. But there have been so many claims about ginseng accomplishing so many different physiological feats that most experts are skeptical. It's true that studies of ginseng in human beings suggest that the herb may slow aging, lengthen life span, and improve performance in long-distance runners and gymnasts, among other things. But none of these studies have been well designed. So we can't say for sure that it was the ginseng that was responsible in each case. On the other hand, these results—although flawed—have led experts to keep an eye on this intriguing herb.

Ginseng is regarded as generally safe, but there are a couple of potential problems. For one thing, ginseng travels through your blood and acts on dif-

pects one thing—back-and-forth or side-to-side motion—but your eyes, ears, and limbs tell the brain something else: movement up, down, and all around.

A study tested ginger on 80 Danish naval cadets who'd not yet gotten their sea legs. Half took 1 gram of ginger in unmarked capsules, the other 40 took look-alike blank capsules. During 4 hours on the open sea, the ginger group reported less cold sweats and vomiting than their mates. And ginger doesn't make you snooze or blur your eyesight, which are common side effects of all motion sickness drugs. Ginger may also help move stomach gas and ease heartburn.

Healing Techniques ▶ Take two 500-milligram capsules of ginger. Or try two or three quarter-sized pieces of crystallized ginger (available commercially). Or put ¼ teaspoon of powdered ginger in a cup of hot water to

ferent parts of your body. This action is presumably responsible for the documented cases of ginseng causing vaginal bleeding in postmenopausal women. And that's not just an annoyance. Vaginal bleeding after menopause may be a warning sign of endometrial cancer. That's not to say ginseng could cause cancer, of course, but it could interfere with the diagnosis.

Also, it seems some people are extremely sensitive to ginseng. If you are, you might get a little jittery and have trouble falling asleep at night (the way you might feel when you're drinking too much coffee). So if you do decide to take ginseng and if you think you're being overstimulated by the herb, stop. Even if you're not sensitive, limit yourself daily to a portion of ginseng root only about the size of your little fingertip.

141

make tea. Take the first dose shortly before your flight or cruise. Repeat every 4 hours, or as needed.

Growing Tips ▶ Plant a ginger root in a large pot with plenty of warmth, moisture, and humidity. Move the pot outdoors in summer. Remove the plant, harvest as much root as you need, then replant it. Dry the root, then grind into powder.

Peppermint

Peppermint calms stomach storms in two ways. It soothes stomach muscles roiled by indigestion, and it frees turbulent gas trapped in your belly by releasing the muscular opening at the top. In other words, it gives you a good burp. Of course, avoid peppermint if you're prone to heartburn from stomach acid escaping into your esophagus.

Peppermint's power has been shown in studies done on people. Now animal-tissue tests are pinning down exactly how peppermint's active ingredient—menthol—does the job. I recommend peppermint tea, even though most digestive aids are "mints." Mints are often made with peppermint flavoring, not with the real McCoy.

By the way, you can use peppermint tea even if you have a stomach ulcer. In fact, it's a safer beverage for you than regular tea or coffee.

Healing Techniques ▶ Steep 1 or 2 teaspoons of peppermint leaf in hot water for several minutes. Sip the tea slowly. You can drink peppermint tea several times a day.

Growing Tips ▶ You should plant peppermint in bottomless plastic pots outdoors to control their rampant roots. Mint plants thrive when set 1 to 1½ feet apart in a partly shady, moist bed.

Special Herbs   17
for Your Heart

Oat bran does, indeed, cut cholesterol, but if you're burning out on oatmeal for breakfast, oat-bran muffins for lunch, and oat-bran fettuccine with oatmeal sauce for dinner, don't despair. Many other foods (beans, broccoli, cauliflower, figs, prunes) and several familiar herbs also reduce cholesterol levels. The best cholesterol-reducing herbs include garlic, ginger, red pepper (cayenne), and fenugreek seed.

Garlic

Garlic is one of the world's oldest medicines. The slaves who built the pyramids received a daily ration to keep them healthy and strong. Garlic is no panacea, but medical journals have published more than a dozen studies confirming the aromatic herb's ability to reduce blood levels of artery-clogging cholesterol. Consider a study published in the British journal *Lancet.* Researchers fed volunteers a high-fat, high-cholesterol meal containing almost 4 ounces of butter. Half the group also consumed 50 grams of garlic juice, the equivalent of eating approximately nine cloves. After 3 hours, cholesterol levels in the no-garlic group had increased 7 percent. But cholesterol levels among the garlic eaters decreased 7 percent. Scientists estimate that every 1 percent decrease in blood cholesterol reduces heart attack risk by about 2 percent, so over time a 7 percent decrease in blood cholesterol levels means a 14 percent drop in the likelihood of a heart attack.

Another study, published in the *American Journal of Clinical Nutrition,* described how volunteers with heart disease and high cholesterol levels ate the equivalent of three cloves of garlic a day for ten months. Compared with controls who ate no garlic, the garlic group's blood cholesterol levels dropped significantly.

Many other human and animal studies have shown similar results. Garlic not only reduces blood cholesterol but also fights heart disease in two other ways oat bran doesn't touch. It reduces blood pressure and inhibits the formation of dangerous arterial blood clots.

The cholesterol-reducing and clot-inhibiting substances in garlic are also found in all the herb's close botanical relatives: onions, scallions, leeks, and chives. Garlic has the most powerful preventive effect, followed by onions, then leeks, scallions, and chives.

Ginger

An old Indian proverb says, "Every good quality is contained in ginger." Like garlic, ginger has been used in herbal medicine since the dawn of history. If you eat this spice only in gingerbread, you're missing a world of flavor. As you enjoy its rich aroma and pungent taste, your arteries will enjoy its ability to reduce cholesterol, demonstrated in a study reported in *Nutrition Reports International*. In addition, ginger reduces blood pressure and blood clotting.

Red Pepper

The fiery taste and bright red appearance of cayenne pepper make it one of the world's most easily noticed spices. But few people have any idea that this spice cuts cholesterol. Red pepper is most widely used in India, where it is an ingredient in many curries. It has also been used in Indian herbal medicine for thousands of years, and modern Indian medical researchers have discovered most of what we know about its biological effects. Two studies—one reported in the *Indian Journal of Experimental Biology,* the other in *Nutrition Reports International*—showed that the chemical responsible for red pepper's heat, capsaicin, has a powerful cholesterol-lowering effect. And like garlic and ginger, red pepper also fights heart disease by inhibiting arterial blood clotting.

If you shy away from red pepper because you grew up believing highly spiced foods cause ulcers, that old saw is now old hat. In a study published in the *Journal of the American Medical Association,* researchers introduced tiny fiberoptic television cameras into subjects' stomachs to get a first-hand look at the effects of hot spices. They concluded that among those with normal digestive systems (that is, no ulcers or ulcerative colitis), even highly spiced foods caused no tissue damage.

Fenugreek Seed

This herb's flavor is a combination of celery and maple. Hippocrates (c. 460–377 B.C.), the Father of Medicine, prescribed a tea made from crushed fenugreek seed for coughs and respiratory ailments. In 19th-century America, the herb was a principal ingredient in Lydia E. Pinkham's Vegetable Compound, a popular patent medicine used to treat menstrual cramps. Fenugreek tea has a soothing quality that may help relieve the dry, hacking cough associated with the common cold, but there's no evidence it treats other respiratory problems or menstrual cramps. However, two studies—one reported in *Current Science* and another in *Atherosclerosis*—showed it produces significant reductions in cholesterol levels.

Ginkgo: An Herb to Keep in Mind   18

The most popular herb in Europe is being prescribed for tinnitus, stroke, and memory loss. Harvey Komet, M.D., of San Antonio, Texas, doesn't have much use for "alternative" medicine. He's an orthodox ear, nose, and throat specialist—and proud of it. But he has started prescribing one herbal medicine—ginkgo.

"My son distributes medicinal herb products for Murdoch Pharmaceuticals, the professional arm of the big herb company, Nature's Way. He knows I treat a good deal of tinnitus [chronic ringing in the ears], and he showed me a tinnitus study by European researchers, who'd obtained good results using ginkgo. Tinnitus is often difficult to treat, so I tried prescribing ginkgo, and got good results. Let me read you this letter from a 60-year-old minister who does missionary work in Mexico. He came in with tinnitus so bad he found it difficult to sleep and concentrate: 'Dear Dr. Komet: I've been taking ginkgo three times a day as you prescribed. It's made a big difference. I still have some ringing, but my ability to think and concentrate has definitely improved. Thank you.'

"His experience is typical. I recommended one 40-milligram tablet three times a day. Quite a few of my tinnitus patients have experienced complete relief. Others, like the minister, have a certain amount of residual ringing, but considerably less than they had before taking ginkgo."

Dr. Komet says he remains "a reluctant ginkgo enthusiast" until well-controlled American studies have replicated the European results his son showed him. "But in my experience, ginkgo is well worthwhile for tinnitus. Several of my patients tell me it also helps with their vertigo. Right now, I'm in the process of setting up a double-blind trial with some people at Tulane and the University of Southern California. We hope to get going in a few months and publish our results by the end of 1991. Ginkgo is a tinnitus treatment people should know about."

Tales of a Healing Herb

Ginkgo, known scientifically as *Ginkgo biloba,* treats more than just tinnitus. Starting about five years ago, American herbalists who visited Europe returned home with stories that sounded like the herbal equivalent of *The Travels of Marco Polo*. There was this exotic herb, ginkgo, they said, and its remarkable healing properties were turning it into a botanical wonder drug in France and Germany. It had proved amazingly effective in treating a broad range of infirmities associated with aging: tinnitus, stroke, memory loss, dizziness (vertigo), one form of hearing loss (cochlear deafness), and age-related vision loss (macular degeneration).

The travelers insisted that ginkgo was being prescribed not only by herbalists but by M.D.'s as well, and that dozens of leading medical research labs were about to publish studies proving the herb's value. Ginkgo tales quickly grew to Paul Bunyan-esque proportions. By 1989, herbalists with European connections were claiming the herb had become the most frequently prescribed medicine in Germany and France.

Of course, terms like "remarkable," "amazing," and "wonder drug" are bandied about alternative medicine frequently—and always turn off the vast majority of mainstream physicians. Most American doctors are skeptical of herbal medicine to begin with and are openly hostile to new herbal discoveries that arrive on the wings of hype. Very few American physicians had ever heard of ginkgo, let alone been impressed by it. And many scientists on this side of the Atlantic have viewed European drug research with considerable suspicion ever since the late 1950s, when a supposedly "safe" European sleep aid, thalidomide, caused severe limb malformations in about 8,000 children of women who took it while pregnant. Those who did not dismiss ginkgo out of hand said they'd wait until the promised studies were published in English.

German Studies Show Results

Then in late 1989, Springer-Verlag, a German scientific publishing company, released an English translation of *Rokan Ginkgo Biloba: Recent Results in Pharmacology and Clinic,* its German anthology of 36 ginkgo

147

studies. (*Rokan* is a German term for ginkgo.) The book was not a best-seller. Unheralded, its tiny press run attracted virtually no attention. It promptly went out of print, and today neither Springer-Verlag's New York office nor other U.S. book distributors have any copies. It's almost as though the ginkgo studies were never published here at all.

But the studies *were* published, and herbalists lucky enough to snap up the compendium began sending ginkgo skeptics photocopies of its many studies. (That's how Dr. Komet first learned of ginkgo. His son sent him a copy of the anthology's tinnitus study.) Anyone who takes even a cursory look at these studies quickly realizes that terms like "remarkable" and "amazing" are right on target—possibly even a bit conservative.

European medical researchers first became excited about ginkgo in the early 1980s, when French scientists showed that it interferes specifically with the action of a substance the body produces called platelet activation factor (PAF). PAF is involved in an enormous number of biological processes, including blood clotting, arterial blood flow, asthma attacks, and organ transplant rejection.

American scientists ignored the French PAF findings, but European researchers jumped into ginkgo experimentation faster than tourists into a new four-star restaurant in Paris. What they discovered has, in just five years, transformed ginkgo from a street tree to Western Europe's leading prescription medicine with sales topping $500 million a year. According to the studies in *Rokan Ginkgo Biloba,* here are just some of ginkgo's benefits.

■ The brain. As people grow older, blood flow in the brain decreases, which means less food and oxygen for brain cells. The findings of William Sneed, M.D., a Venice, California, internist, have confirmed the many European studies showing that ginkgo increases blood flow in the brain, helps prevent and treat stroke, and improves memory and mental prowess.

148
■

■ **The heart.** Ginkgo also improves blood flow to the heart and appears to reduce heart attack risk by preventing the formation of blood clots inside the coronary arteries.

■ **The legs.** When cholesterol deposits narrow the arteries in the legs, the result is "intermittent claudication," pain, cramping, and weakness, particularly in elderly calves. A year-long, double-blind study of 36 intermittent claudication sufferers showed that 40 milligrams of ginkgo three times a day produced "significantly greater relief" than the standard medical treatment.

■ **The eyes.** With age, blood flow decreases to the retina, the nerve-rich area in the back of the eye necessary for sight. As the blood-starved retina deteriorates, the result is "macular degeneration," a leading cause of adult blindness. In a six-month, double-blind French study of ten people with macular degeneration, 80 milligrams of ginkgo twice a day produced "significant vision improvement."

■ **The ears.** With age, blood flow decreases to the nerves of the inner ear necessary for hearing. The result is cochlear deafness, a leading cause of age-related hearing loss. In a 30-day, double-blind French study of 20 people with cochlear deafness, which compared 80 milligrams of ginkgo twice a day with the standard medical therapy, significant recovery was observed in both groups, but improvement was distinctly better in the ginkgo group. Other French studies have shown ginkgo effective in treating tinnitus and vertigo, findings Dr. Komet's observations confirm.

Ginkgo also has other intriguing medical possibilities. Platelet activation factor is involved in triggering asthma attacks. Ginkgo's ability to interfere with PAF may help prevent them. Studies are reportedly now in progress.

Ginkgo is also a powerful antioxidant and free radical scavenger in the bloodstream, which means it may have anticancer effects. Again, no studies have shown this yet, but the American Cancer Society recommends a

149
■

diet high in antioxidant nutrients to help prevent several cancers, particularly colon cancer, the leading cancer killer of nonsmokers.

Finally, preliminary reports from Georgetown University Medical School suggest that a highly purified ginkgo extract (not the commercial extract used in the other ginkgo studies) prevents organ transplant rejection better—and with less toxicity—than the standard anti-rejection drug, cyclosporine. Peter Ramwell, Ph.D., a professor of physiology and biophysics, says he and Marie Foegh, M.D., a professor of surgery, have obtained "very good success" using purified ginkgo extract in experimental heart transplants in rats and lung transplants in dogs. Their research has generated considerable scientific interest because cyclosporine has always been a sharply double-edged therapeutic sword. On the one hand, its rejection-suppression action has helped transform organ transplantation from the laboratory dream it was a generation ago into the major lifesaving industry it is today. But cyclosporine is very expensive and fairly toxic. It often causes kidney problems, high blood pressure, shaking (tremors), and other potentially hazardous side effects.

Meanwhile, ginkgo's only potentially troubling side effect is its anticlotting action. For most people, this is a benefit because it helps prevent heart attack, the nation's leading cause of death. But for those with hemophilia and other clotting disorders, it might be a problem. Nonetheless, compared with cyclosporine, ginkgo is virtually nontoxic.

"If cyclosporine could be replaced by ginkgo," Dr. Ramwell says, "or if the dose of cyclosporine could be reduced with the addition of ginkgo, we'd have a major advance in organ transplantation."

Ancient Asian Medicine

Ginkgo is as poetic as it is promising. It's the oldest surviving tree on earth, and as a medicine it provides the greatest benefits for the oldest surviving people—and anyone who hopes to live to a ripe old age.

A stately tree native to Asia and introduced into the West 250 years ago, ginkgo is the sole survivor of a family of plants related to present-day ferns, which first appeared 200 million years ago during the age of the dinosaurs. Ginkgos grow to 100 feet and have oddly fan-shaped leaves with two lobes (hence the plant's Latin species name, *biloba*), which turn a beautiful golden color before dropping each autumn. Tens of thousands now adorn Buddhist temples across Asia, and streets, parks, and college campuses throughout much of the United States and Europe.

Ginkgo has been used medicinally in Asia since the dawn of history. In China's original herbal, the *Pen Tsao Ching (The Classic of Herbs,* c. 3000 B.C.), the world's first great herbalist, legendary emperor/sage Shen Nung, called it "good for the heart and lungs." Traditional Chinese physicians have used it for thousands of years to treat asthma and other respiratory ailments. Of course, Shen Nung knew nothing of platelet activation factor and its contribution to asthma attacks, but the wise old sage was clearly on to something.

Paul Bergner, editor of the authoritative Portland, Oregon–based newsletter "Medical Herbalism," keeps two ginkgo bonsais on his desk. "I like to commune with them. I'm not sure why, but I feel a spiritual connection with ginkgo that I don't have with too many other herbs. I've even dreamt about ginkgo."

Bergner is all for improvements in organ transplantation, but when he compares U.S. and European ginkgo research, he shakes his head in dismay. "It's so ironic. In Europe, ginkgo is a low-tech plant extract that's become the number one–selling prescription medicine in Germany and France, taken by millions of people for a whole host of infirmities of old age. But here, the only ginkgo research that has received any publicity is the work with organ transplant rejection, a superhigh-tech surgical procedure using a super-purified ginkgo isolate. The

American prejudice in favor of high technology has, in effect, obscured the best uses of this herb, uses that could improve the lives of millions of older Americans."

Consumer Tips

But before you start gobbling ginkgo for its many medical benefits, Bergner has some advice: "Use a 50:1 extract of tannin-free ginkgo with 24 percent flavonoids." This recommendation requires some explanation.

50:1 ▶ "European ginkgo extracts start with 50 pounds of ginkgo leaves and process them into 1 pound of extract, hence 50:1," Bergner explains. "But when the first ginkgo products were marketed in the United States in 1987, the 50:1 extract wasn't available, so the herb companies used an 8:1 extract, which provided a much lower dose. It took a while for some U.S. ginkgo marketers to compensate for this by recommending six times the dose so you'd get the ginkgo equivalent of a 50:1 extract. Meanwhile, 50:1 extracts became available, and herb companies with 50:1 products ran advertisements sniping at the 8:1 products, which confused a lot of people. Now the 50:1 extract has become pretty standard, although some ginkgo tinctures still don't use it. Personally, I recommend 50:1 ginkgo products because that's the European standard. That's the one used in all the studies showing significant benefits."

Tannin-Free ▶ "Like many medicinal herbs, ginkgo leaves contain tannins, astringent chemicals that, in large doses, can cause stomach distress," Bergner says. "When ginkgo products were first introduced in the United States, the tannins were not always removed, and some early users reported often-severe gastrointestinal side effects. Today's 50:1 extracts are tannin-free, but consumers who use other extracts should be aware of the tannin issue and make sure the ginkgo they use is tannin-free."

24 Percent Flavonoids ▶ "Flavonoids are the active chemicals in ginkgo," Bergner explains. "But ginkgo flavonoid content varies depending on what time of year the leaves are harvested. The European studies used extracts with 24 percent flavonoids [or flavone glycosides], and that's become the standard. Look for that on the label when you buy ginkgo."

Bergner says that ginkgo is safe even in large doses but urges the nation's growing number of ginkgo-philes to use the herb cautiously. "In Europe, ginkgo is used primarily to treat age-related ailments in the elderly. These problems require professional care, which is why ginkgo is a prescription drug over there. In this country, ginkgo is sold as an over-the-counter nutritional supplement, and as the word gets out, younger people are using it as a 'brain tonic' to boost intellectual performance and improve memory. I don't see any real harm in that, except possibly expense. Forty milligrams of ginkgo three times a day could run you $40 to $50 a month. And it may take up to six months to get any real effect. On the other hand, there's some recent research support for memory improvement from a single 600-milligram dose. A student cramming for exams might try it—at a cost of about $7.50."

Paul Bergner is no investment adviser, but his ruminations on America's demographic destiny might send stock market speculators scurrying to buy shares in companies that sell ginkgo. "The 77 million baby boomers are entering middle age and getting very nervous about aging, memory loss, and Alzheimer's disease. It's quite possible that 10 or 15 years from now, Americans will be taking ginkgo like they take vitamin C today."

However, Bergner voices mixed emotions about the quality of the ginkgo information now slowly becoming available to the increasingly age-obsessed American public. "On the one hand," he says, "I'd like to see more written about ginkgo because it has the potential to improve the lives of millions of Americans. But I also worry that if the tabloids pick up on ginkgo and blow the re-

153

search out of proportion, the Food and Drug Administration [FDA] might order it off the shelves until someone goes to the tremendous expense of getting it officially licensed."

Some Testimonials

So far, like the vast majority of U.S. physicians, the FDA has shown zero interest in the stately tree that has become literally a "tree of life" for older Europeans. But word has slowly been getting out on this side of the Atlantic, thanks largely to the promotional brochures available where ginkgo products are sold, which summarize the European research. That was how Marie Little, of Miami, Florida, learned of Yerba Prima's ginkgo product, Nutri-Mental.

"My grandmother, age 80, suffers from arthritis, advanced scoliosis [lateral curvature of the spine], and other problems, which have reduced the circulation in her legs," she wrote to Yerba Prima. "Her circulation problem also made her legs feel numb and cold by day and painful at night when she got into bed. She was very uncomfortable and unable to sleep.

"Over the years, as her leg circulation deteriorated, she also developed dark, brownish purple bruises on her legs, which troubled her because they were disfiguring. Her physician told her three years ago that there was nothing he could do to help her legs.

"Then I happened upon your ginkgo pamphlet at my health-food store and thought ginkgo's circulation-promoting effect might help my grandmother. I mentioned it to her, and pretty much out of desperation, she decided to try it. It didn't take long before she noticed improvement in her legs. The numbness, cold, and pain disappeared, and she slept much better. After a few months, the discolored patches on her legs also began to improve.

"My grandmother became very excited and informed her physician about the remarkable improvement in her legs. But instead of sharing her enthusiasm, he simply changed the subject."

Fortunately, when ginkgo comes up, a small but growing number of U.S. physicians don't change the subject. One is Megan Shields, M.D., a West Hollywood, California, family practitioner who has used ginkgo successfully to treat "vascular impotence," a form of erection loss caused by decreased blood flow into the penis.

Dr. Shields says she "never had any interest in alternative medicine" until the late 1970s during her third year of medical school, when she emerged from the classroom and began treating real people. "It didn't take long to see that many of the things the professors taught us should work really didn't work. So I started reading about other forms of healing, and soon realized that mainstream American medicine—allopathy—has no monopoly on cure. I decided I'd be open to whatever works without doing harm. Personally, I still practice allopathic medicine, but I generally take a nutritional approach to healing. I believe it was Hippocrates who said, 'Never give a drug if food will serve.' I don't prescribe pharmaceuticals unless I feel they're absolutely necessary. I also refer people to chiropractors and homeopaths when I think they might help."

One way Dr. Shields keeps up with nutritional medicine is by reading *The Townsend Letter for Doctors,* an offbeat medical journal published in Port Townsend, Washington, which scours the scientific literature to find credible research validating alternative healing arts. In late 1989, *The Townsend Letter* reported the results of a ginkgo study published earlier that year in *The Journal of Urology.* That study, which the mass media greeted with a thundering silence, is the first ginkgo study to appear in a U.S. medical journal. The researchers recruited 60 men with vascular erection loss who had not responded to the standard medical treatment, papaverine, an opium derivative that opens the arteries and often increases blood flow into the penis. The men took 50 milligrams of ginkgo a day for 12 to 18 months. Half regained their erections, and another 20 percent subsequently responded to a combination of ginkgo and papaverine. The researchers concluded: "Ginkgo appears to be very effective in the treatment of arterial erectile dysfunction."

Dr. Shields had never heard of ginkgo before, but shortly after she read the Townsend report, an otherwise healthy 60-year-old man consulted her for erection loss. "Impotence has many possible causes," Dr. Shields explains, "but it takes a major medical workup with lots of tests to zero in on the cause. This man was quite healthy and didn't have any of the problems that often cause erection loss—diabetes, depression, alcoholism, and relationship problems. I suspected a vascular problem, but to figure out what was going on, I told him he'd need a battery of tests. Then I mentioned the ginkgo study and asked if he'd like to try it before having the big workup. He said ginkgo sounded worth trying, so I sent him down to the local health-food store. Within three weeks, he could have erections again."

Since then, Dr. Shields has prescribed ginkgo to two other men with erection loss. "In all three cases, the ginkgo worked within three weeks. Of course, my results are anecdotal. Maybe my three patients were just lucky. Maybe the combination of my touting ginkgo and the patients' belief in it had some placebo effect. Who knows? All I know is that ginkgo is harmless, and affordable, and it worked. It saved my patients a good deal of time, trouble, and trauma in workups they didn't need. Next time someone comes to me for what looks like a possible vascular erection problem, you better believe I'm going to see if they respond to ginkgo."

But when asked if her work with ginkgo has extended beyond vascular impotence to its many other therapeutic benefits, Dr. Shields said she was unaware of any other uses. "What? Are you serious? Ginkgo helps prevent and treat stroke? It improves intellectual performance? It treats tinnitus? No kidding. That's amazing. I had no idea. Do you have those studies? Would you send them to me? I want to learn all about ginkgo."

The
Frontiers
of
Medical
Care

19   Arthritis Treatments
of Tomorrow

If you detect arthritis in its early stages, what hope do you have of nipping it in the bud—of actually stopping it before it gets worse? Or if you can't catch it early, what hope is there of stopping it at all?

The answer used to be: none. But now preliminary research hints that there may be a chance to do the impossible after all: to halt the pain, joint damage, and inflammation. And not just for a few hours or days, but for good. This hope hinges on factors like an arthritis "vaccination," which, if confirmed in studies, could revolutionize treatment.

Here's a closer look at some of these promising anti-arthritis strategies.

Killing an Arthritis Bug

Some fascinating research suggests that a large number of cases (maybe as many as 2,000 a year) of inflammatory arthritis may be caused by the body's reaction to a bacterial infection, such as Lyme disease. In targeting the infection, the immune system also causes arthritic inflammation in the joints. If this is so, then treatment with the proper antibiotic might correct the problem at the source rather than merely relieve the symptoms.

Minnesota physician Erskine M. Caperton, M.D., and his colleagues tested this hypothesis on 59 people with different forms of inflammatory arthritis. All 59 also had antibody evidence of a bacterial infection. The bacterium has been associated with Lyme disease, a malady that can cause chronic inflammatory arthritis.

Thirty-nine of the patients received the antibiotic

ceftriaxone; 20 of them got a placebo. After two weeks of treatment, 19 of the 39 patients getting the antibiotic had improved in symptoms like tender joints, fatigue, and morning stiffness. Only 2 of the 20 placebo patients showed improvement.

"In some patients the response was spectacular," says Dr. Caperton. "One 72-year-old woman had severe, chronic, nodular rheumatoid . . . arthritis that was incapacitating for 18 months. Because of a strongly positive Lyme antibody test, she had been treated with tetracycline and with penicillin intravenously without improvement. . . . Following ceftriaxone, she reduced her prednisone [an anti-inflammatory drug] from 15 milligrams per day to none, regained mobility, and resumed normal activity." The woman's number of tender joints fell from 70 to 18, and her swollen joints from 36 to 12. Seven months after receiving therapy, her arthritis returned, but not as severely as before the ceftriaxone.

These results do not mean that all arthritis patients are actually suffering from the latent effects of Lyme disease or some other bacterial infection, says Arthur Grayzel, M.D., senior vice-president for medical affairs of the Arthritis Foundation. Nor does it mean that all arthritis patients should ask their doctor for this antibiotic.

"Inflammatory arthritis is one of the acute manifestations of Lyme disease," Dr. Grayzel says. "And the arthritis is usually quite responsive to antibiotics when they're used within the first several months after infection. Once the arthritis has gone on for several years, then it's not clear that treating the organism is sufficient.

"There isn't much theoretical reason for assuming that antibiotics would be useful in treating other forms of inflammatory arthritis, such as rheumatoid arthritis. This is the sort of study that needs confirmation with other research using very tight controls. Only then can we know for sure whether bacteria can cause other kinds of arthritis."

In the meantime, Dr. Grayzel says it would be a good idea for people who live in areas where Lyme disease is common and who have arthritis and have not been tested for Lyme disease to talk to their physicians about it.

Better Than Gold

There was a time when the best and brightest hope for dampening down arthritis symptoms was injections of gold salts. The gold treatment can sometimes ease symptoms for long periods, essentially putting the disease into remission. But gold injections cause very serious side effects. Along came oral gold, which had much milder side effects but much less power to halt symptoms.

Enter methotrexate (MTX). This is the newest and most promising of the so-called disease-modifying anti-rheumatic drugs (DMARDs). Several studies have shown that in rheumatoid arthritis, MTX can dramatically slow the disease process, ease symptoms, and help patients reduce steroid doses. And side effects of the drug are proving to be easier to live with than those of other DMARDs.

"MTX's biggest advantage over other DMARDs is its fast action," says Walter G. Barr, M.D., chief of rheumatology at Loyola University Medical Center in Chicago. "With other DMARDs, you'd have to wait three to four months before you would see results. And you may not get results with the first one you tried, so you'd have to wait another three to four months. MTX starts working in four to six weeks."

In all previous research, MTX was shown to work in people who had already been treated unsuccessfully with other DMARDs, including gold. So some researchers wondered if MTX would work in people who hadn't been treated with any DMARD. To find out, they recently tested 281 people with active, adult-onset rheumatoid arthritis. For nine months, about half of the people got MTX and half got oral gold. At the end of the study, the MTX patients had fewer painful joints, fewer swollen joints, less pain, and less morning stiffness than those patients getting the oral gold.

What's more, many of the side effects that are common to DMARDs (gastrointestinal problems, rash, headache) were much less prevalent in those taking MTX.

Because of such good study results, a lot of doctors have started prescribing MTX.

Getting the Light Treatment

Imagine someday "vaccinating" rheumatoid arthritis patients and putting their bodies' immune systems to work destroying the cells responsible for the inflammation and pain of the disease and slowing or stopping the disease process. You may not have to imagine this treatment too much longer, for medical researchers across the country are testing it in clinical trials right now.

This experimental treatment, called photopheresis, combines a light-sensitive drug with a high-tech machine and ultraviolet light to selectively modify the disease-producing cells so the immune system can better identify and destroy them.

Dr. Barr, whose Loyola University Medical Center is one of the centers participating in the national trials, says that the treatment is based on the knowledge that abnormal T-cells from the immune system are involved in rheumatoid arthritis.

"We know that T-cells are important to the disease," says Dr. Barr, "because if you look at the synovial lining [tissue surrounding the joints] in an arthritic, you'll see increased numbers of T-cells. If you remove T-cells from the blood, the patient will improve."

Dr. Barr and his colleagues administer the drug 8-methoxypsoralen (8-MOP), a medication that works only when activated by exposure to ultraviolet-A light. Next a machine pumps blood out of your arm and, before returning it to the other arm, separates it into red cells and white cells. Then the machine exposes the white cells, including the abnormal T-cells containing 8-MOP, to ultraviolet-A light. Once activated, 8-MOP modifies the T-cells in such a way that the immune system recognizes

161

them as harmful and destroys them. Other cells are not affected.

Photopheresis has already been used successfully in two serious diseases involving renegade T-cells: T-cell lymphoma, a deadly form of leukemia, and scleroderma, an arthritis-like disease. A very early pilot study using photopheresis in rheumatoid arthritis resulted in an impressive decrease in the number of swollen and painful joints in four out of seven patients.

Although this study is small, researchers are excited about the results, because T-cell vaccinations are a whole new approach to therapy. T-cell vaccinations have already been shown to work in animals. And amazingly enough, the treatment is essentially nontoxic. Its nearest kin—the broad-spectrum immune-suppressing drugs for rheumatoid arthritis—carries severe side effects. The drugs kill good cells and bad, so people can end up with recurrent infections, among other things.

"The real question is how long-lasting the benefit is," says Dr. Grayzel. "This research looks promising, but they've treated only a small number of people. There's a lot of work to be done before it gets applied in a widespread fashion to rheumatoid arthritis. Nevertheless, this is definitely something that is under active investigation."

How long will it be before photopheresis is adequately tested and widely available for arthritis patients? The treatment is currently approved by the Food and Drug Administration (FDA) only for treatment of T-cell lymphoma. An appeal is before the FDA for approval for its use in scleroderma. Dr. Barr estimates that the nationwide study will be complete in a year or so. If the results prove that the process is effective, we will be much closer to wider availability of photopheresis.

Not Just a Pain in the Chest

If you're one of the 1.5 million Americans who will have a heart attack this year, there's something important you should know.

You can cut your risk of dying of a heart attack in half if you get to the hospital within an hour of feeling the first twinge of pain. Some experts believe you can lower your risk even further by popping an aspirin under your tongue (or swallowing it) while awaiting help.

Unfortunately, many people do nothing and wait, either ignoring their symptoms or writing them off as indigestion or muscle spasm. According to national studies, about half of all heart attack victims wait up to 2 hours to seek medical help. During that critical time, many die. Those who are lucky enough to survive suffer irreparable damage to their heart.

But lives can be saved and heart damage minimized thanks to a family of drugs that are widely known by a name that makes them sound more like a Saturday morning cartoon than lifesaving medication. They're called "clot busters."

If administered within an hour of the onset of symptoms, clot busters, or thrombolytic agents, can stop a heart attack in its tracks. They work by dissolving blood clots that block the flow of blood and oxygen to the heart—the cause of the majority of heart attacks. Usually about a half hour into an attack, some of the heart muscle is irreparably damaged. But the clot busters clear the blood vessels rapidly, protecting areas of the heart not yet affected by the heart attack. Damage to and deterioration of the heart muscle, which would affect how the heart works, is minimized. Clot-busting drugs are very effective. Doctors are able to clear arteries with clot blockage in 75 to 80 percent of patients.

But the key to the clot busters' success is that they

must be administered rapidly after onset of symptoms. As time passes and more of the heart muscle is damaged, their effectiveness drops off dramatically, although they still have a "salvaging effect" 4 to 6 hours after the onset of a heart attack—if you survive it. However, some studies suggest that even up to 24 hours there may be some benefit.

"But the patient needs to react much sooner," says Peter Barath, M.D., research scientist in cardiology at Cedars–Sinai Medical Center in California. "From our experience, about 50 percent of heart attack victims die within an hour of the onset of symptoms, before they reach the hospital. The patient needs to get to the hospital within that hour."

Why Wait?

Why do so many heart attack victims wait to report pain that in some cases feels like "an elephant sitting on your chest," in the words of one survivor? According to a study conducted by Andreas T. J. Wielgosz, M.D., Ph.D., of the University of Ottawa, procrastinating heart attack victims give four reasons: They believe they are invulnerable; they misinterpret warning signals; they try to treat themselves (e.g., by taking an antacid for "indigestion"); or they suffer in silence. They simply don't believe they're having a heart attack.

It's not unusual for people to mistake milder heart attack pains for indigestion or even muscle spasms. About one-eighth of heart attacks are so-called silent heart attacks, with no apparent symptoms. And there are some people who are just plain embarrassed that they might be rushing into the hospital for an acute bellyache.

But it doesn't make sense to die of embarrassment. What does make sense is to pay attention to unusual symptoms. And seek medical treatment at once, particularly if you are at high risk for a heart attack, either because of a genetic predisposition or lifestyle reasons (you're overweight, have high blood pressure, high blood cholesterol, smoke, are a man, or are over 65).

How do you know if you're having a heart attack? Since warning signals vary, you may not. But it's better to be diagnosed with gastritis than delay getting help for a heart attack.

Generally, heart attack pain is not just a nagging, fleeting pain. It's an uncomfortable, lasting pain that does not disappear after 10 minutes. You may feel pressure, tightness, squeezing, heaviness, or very infrequently, a pain in your chest, which may radiate to your back, shoulders, neck, arms, and even fingers. It may be accompanied by light-headedness, sweating, nausea, vomiting, and shortness of breath.

While pain relieved by food or antacids probably is indigestion or ulcers, pain brought on by exertion and relieved by rest is usually a sign of heart disease. If you experience these symptoms, call your doctor at once. At the very least, tell someone how you feel. In his study, Dr. Wielgosz found that when a heart attack victim told someone about chest pain, there was less delay in getting to a hospital.

Follow your doctor's instructions. If you need to be admitted to a hospital, never drive yourself. Call for a paramedic if no one else can drive you. In fact, you might want to call the paramedics right away. In some parts of the country, paramedics can administer thrombolytic agents with a doctor's permission.

Although it may sound impossible, try to relax while you wait. Loosen your belt, tie, or collar, which may help you to breathe easier. Take some deep breaths. Although half a million people die of heart attacks every year, a heart attack doesn't have to be a killer. But, according to some experts, panic can be. (See "Having a Heart Attack? Relax" on page 166.)

Clot-Busting Decisions

Before administering a clot-busting drug, a doctor must examine your medical history. Not everyone is a good candidate for thrombolytic agents, for several reasons, including age, allergies, how quickly you get to the

165
■

HAVING A HEART ATTACK? RELAX

It's easier said than done. But if you're having a heart attack, the best thing you can do—after calling for help—is to relax. You may survive the heart attack if you don't let panic kill you.

When Norman Cousins had a heart attack in 1980, he stayed calm. And to minimize the stress of the situation, the former editor of *Saturday Review* and author of *The Healing Heart* asked the driver of his ambulance to turn off the siren and drive at an ordinary speed.

Not only does panic make a heart attack harder to deal with psychologically, it takes its toll physically, too, by aggravating the heart's weakened condition and making it work harder. According to Herbert Benson, M.D., a Harvard Medical School associate professor and cardiologist at New England Deaconess Hospital, Boston, panic increases the amount of catecholamines in the body. Catecholamines—also known as the adrenalines—are epinephrine and norepinephrine. They make the heart beat faster, blood pressure rise, and blood clot more quickly—effects you don't want when the heart is already trying to compensate for the lack of oxygen caused by a blood clot or other obstacle.

hospital, and more. Unfortunately, there is a risk involved—a chance the drugs may stimulate internal bleeding or cause a stroke. Since the purpose of the medication is to get blood flowing, the risk of bleeding is a direct result, not a side effect, of the breaking up (thrombolysis) of a blood clot.

If you have previously had a stroke, if you have an active bleeding disorder, such as a bleeding ulcer, hemorrhoids, or hemophilia, or if you have excessive high blood pressure, you're probably not a good candidate for

Rather than putting unnecessary stress on your heart, try to relax by using some of the principles of the relaxation response laid out in a book by the same name by Dr. Benson. After calling for medical assistance and taking nitroglycerine (if prescribed), try the four-step process for relaxation.

- Sit quietly.
- Sit comfortably.
- Focus on a stimulus, such as a mental image or a calming word, repeated in your mind.
- Disregard intruding thoughts that disturb your relaxation.

Says John Deckro, R.N., of the New England Deaconess Hospital, "You can achieve a state of rest, which can reverse the effects of the stress hormones and actually can work to decrease the demand for oxygen in the heart."

Sounds tough under the circumstances, but in the long run, simple relaxation could be just the ticket for making it through your heart attack safely.

thrombolysis. Other bleeding risk factors are recent surgery or accident, advancing age, head trauma, and active ulcer.

The doctor will also want to analyze your symptoms and run an electrocardiogram (EKG) to confirm that you are in fact having a heart attack. An EKG records the heart's electrical impulses and picks up the abnormal impulses that signal a heart attack. About 50 percent of patients have a classic EKG reading, meaning the results show an unquestionable heart attack. For those whose

EKG is not so well defined, an ultrasound can sometimes be performed to remove doubt about how the heart is functioning.

Sometimes a doctor administers a thrombolytic medication in cases that are not clear-cut, as long as the risk of bleeding or stroke is minimal. Even in heart attacks that aren't caused by blood clots—about 15 percent are caused by the contraction or spasm of an artery—your physician may decide to give you a clot buster anyway. The drug may ensure that a new clot doesn't form and cause complications, says Daniel Shindler, M.D., assistant professor of medicine at the Robert Wood Johnson Medical School in New Brunswick, New Jersey.

Clot busters have been in use for over 20 years. Until 1988 they were used in conjunction with angioplasty, a procedure not every hospital performs. Since then, a study has shown that the drugs are as effective alone as when followed by angioplasty. Now clot busters can be given in almost any emergency room, not just in hospitals equipped for balloon angioplasty. "That's the beauty of the medicine. It can be administered in any emergency room equipped to handle coronary patients," says Dr. Shindler. "The idea is just to get to the closest one fast."

Take Your Pick

Three clot busters that have been approved by the Food and Drug Administration are available. Tissue plasminogen activator (t-PA) is administered intravenously over a 3-hour period with heparin, a blood thinner. Heparin is given intravenously toward the end of the t-PA infusion while t-PA is still active in the bloodstream. You may also be given aspirin with these clot busters, to keep clots from coming back over the longer term. Aspirin is also used in conjunction with streptokinase, another clot buster, which is administered over a 1-hour period and lasts in the circulation for about an hour. There has been some controversy recently over which of these two clot-busting drugs works better. Results of studies comparing the effectiveness of t-PA versus streptokinase vary widely. While one study showed them to be similarly effective in saving lives, critics claim t-PA is quicker acting and far more effective. They also point out that the drug heparin was not used correctly in the trial that proved the two of equal effectiveness. Both t-PA and streptokinase are short-acting drugs, given by IV over a long period of time because the medication doesn't remain in the bloodstream for long.

Antistreplase (APSAC), the newest clot buster, is a longer-acting drug. And an ongoing international study is expected to rate its effectiveness compared to that of the two older medications. Unlike t-PA and streptokinase, APSAC can be administered by simple intravenous injection in 2 to 5 minutes. It lasts about 24 hours.

The clot busters vary greatly in price. Streptokinase can cost up to $400 a dose, while t-PA runs up to $2,200. APSAC falls somewhere in between, at about $1,000. Costs may be covered by insurance.

Clot busters aren't a cure-all, however. Most of the time, partial blockage in the artery remains in the form of cholesterol plaque, says Jeffrey Anderson, M.D., chief of the Cardiology Division at Intermountain Heart Institute, Salt Lake City. Additional measures, such as surgery or angioplasty, may be considered.

But according to cardiologist Dean Ornish, M.D., director of the Preventive Medicine Research Institute, drugs like clot busters should be the beginning rather than the end of recovery from heart disease. "All too often," he says, "a patient survives the heart attack and then goes back to doing the same things that led to the heart problems in the first place."

Dr. Ornish thinks recovery requires not only thrombolysis but also a complete change of lifestyle to one that emphasizes stress management, moderate exercise, and a low-fat diet as described in his book *Dr. Dean Ornish's Program for Reversing Heart Disease*. After all, the best way to survive a heart attack may be to avoid becoming a candidate for another one.

21   Is Your Thyroid out of Whack?

America's First Lady described it better than any doctor could have. "My thyroid gland just went wacko," Barbara Bush explained after she'd been diagnosed as having Graves' disease, a potentially serious condition in which the thyroid pumps out excess amounts of hormone.

Barbara Bush is certainly in good company. She's one of about seven million Americans known to have a thyroid disorder. Another three million have a problem thyroid but don't know it. In fact, thyroid disorders occur much more often than even many doctors realize. They're particularly common among middle-aged and older women, where they often go unrecognized or are often mistaken for something else.

The butterfly-shaped thyroid gland is in the neck, its two wings wrapped around the windpipe just below the Adam's apple. The thyroid weighs less than an ounce, but it can have an enormous impact on your health.

Think of it as the body's regulator. It does the job by releasing two hormones, the more important of which is the iodine-containing hormone thyroxine. The hormones help regulate heartbeat, body temperature, how quickly a person burns calories, how swiftly food moves through the digestive tract, and more.

Normally, the thyroid doles out just the right amount of hormone to keep these processes humming smoothly. But it may turn overactive and pump out too much hormone, or underactive and pump out too little. Either way, the abnormal hormone level can profoundly affect the body's metabolism.

In the Slow Lane

Probably five million Americans have an underactive thyroid, a condition called hypothyroidism, the most common thyroid problem. In most cases, it's caused by an autoimmune reaction. No one knows exactly why, but the immune system makes antibodies that mistakenly attack and damage thyroid cells, progressively reducing the thyroid's hormone output.

Hypothyroidism causes all the body's processes to slow down. Yet many people with underactive thyroids don't know it. The American Thyroid Association estimates that half of all people with hypothyroidism haven't been diagnosed, or they've been misdiagnosed.

For unknown reasons, hypothyroidism overwhelmingly afflicts women, especially those between 35 and 60. They develop the condition four times more often than men. Some experts recommend a thyroid examination as part of every gynecological checkup.

In a thyroid exam, the doctor carefully feels the thyroid gland to see if it's abnormally enlarged. An enlarged thyroid, known as a goiter, can occur in both hyperthyroidism and hypothyroidism. If you do have a goiter, your doctor can then order blood tests to determine the cause of the thyroid problem.

Compared to other diseases, hypothyroidism can be difficult to recognize, especially in older people. Unless doctors suspect a thyroid problem, they may mistake the varied symptoms for psychosomatic complaints or attribute them to normal female aging.

The woman herself is often fooled, too. Hypothyroidism usually comes on gradually, over several months or even years. The early clues may be scarcely noticeable, or you may attribute them to other causes. You may feel tired most of the time, have weak or aching muscles, feel cold, be constipated, or gain weight even though you're eating less.

As the thyroid continues losing steam, you may notice that your face looks puffier or your hair looks coarse. Your nails may be brittle, and your skin may seem drier than usual. Or you may notice that a necklace that once hung loosely now feels like a choker. Your thyroid has grown bigger, developing into a goiter, as it attempts to manufacture more hormone.

171

(In past decades, people often developed goiters because they lived in parts of the country where food and water lacked iodine, which the thyroid must have to make its hormones. Now that iodine is added to salt, iodine deficiency is rarely a cause of hypothyroidism.)

Other physical symptoms of hypothyroidism include cramps, dizziness, a deepening voice, and abnormal menstrual periods—quite heavy or absent. Hypothyroidism may also increase blood cholesterol levels. Some experts now recommend testing people with high cholesterol levels to see if their thyroid is a contributing factor.

And then there are the effects that hypothyroidism can have on mental functioning: inability to concentrate, forgetfulness, and depression. These mental symptoms have led to tragic cases where hypothyroidism was misdiagnosed as senility, madness, or psychosis, says Steven R. Gambert, M.D., chairman of geriatrics and gerontology at New York Medical College.

"Signs and symptoms of hypothyroidism are more easily recognized in a 20-year-old patient," Dr. Gambert says. "Unfortunately, in a 70-year-old, these same signs and symptoms are too often dismissed as accompaniments of ordinary aging." He recommends that doctors determine if a failing thyroid could be the real cause of their older patients' problems.

Fortunately, doctors can easily diagnose hypothyroidism with new and sensitive blood tests. And once the problem is diagnosed, treatment is as simple as a once-a-day tablet. The tablet contains thyroid hormone to compensate for the thyroid's diminished output. Like a fresh rewind for a run-down clock, the replacement therapy primes a sluggish metabolism.

All Revved Up

Picture yourself sitting in a car that's idling quietly in the driveway, until you press the accelerator to the floor. About two million Americans are similarly revved up. Their thyroid pumps out excess hormones, which push their metabolism into overdrive. This is hyperthyroidism, and it may produce diverse symptoms: frequent loose stools, heightened sensitivity to heat, excessive sweating, weight loss, fatigue, muscle weakness, nervousness, irritability, insomnia, and hand tremors. Another symptom—a rapidly pounding heart when you're at rest—can be especially serious. It can intensify chest pain in people with heart disease and even cause a heart attack.

Barbara Bush lost 18 pounds in two months without dieting—a classic sign of hyperthyroidism. She also developed eye problems. In her words, they started getting "big, puffy, horrible." That was the tip-off to Graves' disease, named after a 19th-century Irish physician. It's the most common type of hyperthyroidism, accounting for half of all cases. And it can be fatal if left untreated.

Graves' disease affects mainly women, especially those ages 30 to 55. Like hypothyroidism, it's an autoimmune disease. In Graves' disease, some antibodies attack thyroid cells, stimulating them to produce excess amounts of hormones. Other antibodies may attack the muscles and other tissues around the eye. As these tissues become inflamed, they push against the eyeball and cause the symptoms that bothered Mrs. Bush: bulging of the eyeball, painful pressure, and persistent double vision. The pressure can lead to blindness if it's not corrected.

Treating Graves' disease may require treating both the thyroid gland and the eyes. That's what happened with Mrs. Bush. In fact, the steps her doctors took in treating her provide a good illustration.

People diagnosed with Graves' disease are usually started on antithyroid medication—drugs that stop overproduction of thyroid hormones. These drugs are taken until the disease goes into remission, says Leonard Wartofsky, M.D., chief of the Endocrine-Metabolic Service at Walter Reed Army Medical Center, where Mrs. Bush was treated. "We try to determine whether their hyperthyroidism may go into remission during drug treatment within a reasonable period of time—usually 6 to 18 months."

Methimazole, the antithyroid drug prescribed for Mrs. Bush, is often the only treatment that patients

173

need. When remission doesn't occur, further therapy is necessary.

"In older patients, our first concern is always their cardiac status," Dr. Wartofsky explains. "Hyperthyroidism may impose considerable stress on the heart. In such patients, we're more likely to abandon antithyroid drugs earlier and progress to radioactive iodine therapy of the thyroid."

That was the treatment course in Mrs. Bush's case. To permanently cool her overactive thyroid, Mrs. Bush drank a solution of radioactive iodine. The hormone-producing cells of the thyroid absorb the iodine and are killed by the radioactivity. The result: a defunct thyroid. Sounds drastic, but radioactive iodine has been a standard hyperthyroid treatment for more than 50 years. The iodine is trapped in the thyroid or is excreted by the kidneys, destroying thyroid cells without damaging other tissues or causing side effects. The resulting underfunctioning thyroid gland can then be easily corrected with daily doses of replacement hormone.

The iodine treatment and thyroid hormone failed to solve Mrs. Bush's eye problems, however. To treat the inflammation that was causing these problems, doctors first tried large doses of steroids. But long-term steroid use can cause serious side effects, including softened bones and diabetes. So Mrs. Bush began a series of ten treatments in which low-dose radiation beams are aimed at her eyes. This procedure is not always an option. But when it is indicated, and performed properly, it is painless and complications are minimal. The radiation beams are targeted at the swollen tissue behind the eyes, avoiding the eyeballs themselves. The radiation should help relieve the pressure that's causing her eyes to bulge and reduce the inflammation of her eye muscles that's causing her double vision.

Getting the Right Medicine

174
∎

Whatever your thyroid problem, chances are you take thyroid hormone to treat it. In hypothyroidism, thyroid hormone restores metabolism to normal. And most people diagnosed with hyperthyroidism ultimately take thyroid hormone, too. As with Mrs. Bush, their thyroid often is purposely knocked out of action, which results in hypothyroidism; normal levels of hormone are then restored by a daily thyroid hormone tablet.

More people take thyroid hormone for other thyroid maladies. Since these occur mainly in women, it's not surprising that thyroid hormone ranks as one of the drugs that women take most often.

Once a woman starts taking thyroid hormone, she usually takes it every day for the rest of her life. With this kind of long-term therapy, a drug should produce consistent effects. That's why a synthetic thyroid hormone is much preferred over the older, natural variety.

Today's thyroid medicine of choice is levothyroxine sodium. This newer, man-made version of natural thyroid hormone costs only about 15 cents a day.

But unfortunately, not everyone uses the synthetic type. A study published in the *Journal of the American Medical Association* found that many older people still take the natural kind, obtained from the thyroid glands of slaughtered animals. But in this case, "natural" may not be as healthy as synthetic. The thyroid hormone obtained from animals is unpredictable. The kind of animals used, what they ate, the season they were slaughtered—all can cause the hormone's potency to vary from one batch to another.

By contrast, the synthetic variety is pure, standardized from batch to batch, and identical in chemical structure to human thyroid hormone. Many doctors have switched their patients from natural to synthetic thyroid, and some believe that all patients should switch.

"There is no longer a role for animal thyroid in the treatment of hypothyroidism," says Dr. Gambert. He's particularly concerned about the many elderly patients who've been taking animal thyroid for years, and who often are no longer under a doctor's care. Dr. Gambert urges them to contact their doctor to get their medication reassessed. If you're taking animal thyroid, ask your doc-

175
■

tor if synthetic thyroid might be a better choice. No one should take any hormone preparation without consulting a doctor.

There's also good reason to have yourself rechecked if you've been on thyroid hormones. Until about 1960, doctors believed that a sluggish thyroid caused many common maladies. Lacking accurate thyroid function tests, doctors prescribed thyroid hormone on a hunch rather than with solid evidence that patients needed it. So it's possible that some people who haven't checked with their doctor since getting a prescription long ago for thyroid hormone may be taking the medication for nothing.

It's now known that thyroid hormone should be used only for specific disorders, such as hypothyroidism, benign goiter, thyroid nodule, and cancer of the thyroid. Taking unnecessary thyroid probably isn't dangerous for most people, but it's risky for some. If you're on thyroid medication but think you might not need it, don't discontinue therapy on your own. You can withdraw safely, but only under a doctor's care.

Getting the Right Dose

Doctors take special care to prescribe the minimal effective dose of thyroid hormone for people with a weak heart—some elderly persons and others at risk for coronary artery disease. For these people, excess thyroid hormone may cause a heart attack or worsen coronary artery disease. Now evidence suggests that doctors should take the same care when administering thyroid to other patients: women, young and old.

Until recently, long-term treatment with thyroid hormone was considered relatively safe. Doctors didn't worry much about giving more hormone than the woman needed, as long as it didn't produce symptoms of hyperthyroidism.

In the past few years, however, studies have shown that too much replacement thyroid hormone may increase a woman's risk for osteoporosis, the bone-thinning disorder that can lead to fractures of the hip and vertebrae.

One of those studies appeared in the *Journal of the American Medical Association.* The study involved two groups of women: 31 premenopausal women who'd been receiving levothyroxine for more than five years and 31 other women of the same age and weight, who weren't taking thyroid medication. Using a special technique, doctors measured the hipbone densities of women in both groups.

The women being treated with thyroid hormone had significantly lower hipbone densities than women not on thyroid. The differences were most striking in women over 35. The scientists reported that many of the subjects were receiving doses of thyroid hormone that would now be considered excessive.

"When using thyroxine therapeutically, one must choose the dosage with great care," says David S. Cooper, M.D., an endocrinologist at Johns Hopkins University School of Medicine. Dr. Cooper warns that a large number of patients face an increased risk of bone loss because their dose of thyroid hormone is too high. Luckily, there's now a way to pinpoint the optimum dose.

Getting the Right Test

Until recently, doctors lacked a sensitive test of thyroid function—a way to gauge if the gland was overactive or underactive and by how much. But now a sophisticated test can diagnose thyroid problems that have gone unrecognized in the past. And it allows doctors to gauge the optimum dose of replacement thyroid hormone that best suits each patient's needs.

The old thyroid function test measures blood levels of the main thyroid hormone, thyroxine. But a wide range of thyroxine levels can be considered "normal." A "low-normal" reading may be okay for one person's metabolism but too skimpy for another's. Using a highly sensitive technique, the new test measures a different hormone, thyroid stimulating hormone, or TSH.

TSH comes from the pituitary gland and does what its name suggests: stimulates the thyroid to release its hormone. The pituitary sends out TSH in response to the amount of thyroid hormone it senses in the blood. A high TSH level tells you the thyroid isn't making enough hormone.

Normal TSH levels vary less than normal levels of thyroid hormone, making TSH values easier to interpret. A low thyroxine reading, for example, suggests—but doesn't prove—that you have hypothyroidism. Using the new TSH test, your doctor may not need to do other blood tests; a high TSH level confirms that hypothyroidism is present. And in most cases, the test can detect both hypothyroidism and hyperthyroidism.

If you think you have a thyroid disorder, the American Thyroid Association recommends that you ask your doctor for a TSH blood test.

The TSH test can also help the three million Americans already on thyroid therapy. Their need for replacement hormone may change over the years. An annual TSH test lets doctors fine-tune your dose, giving enough for normal metabolism but not an excess that could increase osteoporosis risk.

For free information on thyroid problems, write to the Thyroid Foundation of America, Inc., Massachusetts General Hospital, ACC7305, Boston, MA 02114. To locate a qualified thyroid specialist near you, call the American Thyroid Association, Walter Reed Army Medical Center, Washington, D.C., at (202) 882-7717.

22 At the Cutting Edge of Medical Treatment

"Better than the best" is the kind of phrase that makes the brain's skepticism meter hop, skip, and jump off the chart. Sometimes, however, you really can get something that's better than the best when it comes to medical treatment—if you're enrolled in a clinical trial. Clinical trials are scientific tests of new treatments.

And some trials offer you the chance to get a new drug, device, or surgical technique that's at least as good as the best standard treatment . . . and that maybe, just maybe, might turn out to be better than the standard. The right clinical trial could very well be an offer you don't want to refuse.

Catch a Rising Star

As your eyes scan this line, scientists and researchers around the world are testing new and possibly better treatments for a variety of ailments. These tests are a weeding-out process: Only a handful of potential new treatments are adopted as standard therapies. Most drugs are first tested in a laboratory against microorganisms or cell cultures. That's known as an in vitro (*in VEE troh;* Latin for "in glass") trial. The next step is in vivo (*in VEE voh;* Latin for "in life") testing, performed on laboratory animals. Many new drugs and medical devices (artificial heart valves, for example) and ground-breaking surgical procedures are first tested at this level. Drugs that have shown promise in vitro often move on to in vivo tests in more than one species of animal when necessary.

When enough promising evidence has been gathered, doctors interested in conducting clinical trials apply to the Food and Drug Administration (FDA) for an investigational new drug application (IND), or an investigational device exemption (IDE). Each of these is basically a safety review before initial testing in humans. In addition, each hospital and research center must have the details of any proposed clinical trial approved by the Institutional Review Board, which acts as a stern advocate for patients' rights and safety.

In drug testing, there are three levels of testing done in humans to objectively prove the value of a new drug while identifying and controlling possible side effects. Phase I trials are performed with low doses on a small number of people (usually 20 to 200) to learn how this drug acts in humans, its potential side effects, and opti-

179
■

mum dosage. Phase II trials are usually performed on from 50 to several hundred people: Usually, half are given the new drug and half are given a placebo (an inactive substance that looks like the new drug) or a currently approved product.

The purpose of Phase II trials is to test the effectiveness of a dosage range in an objective manner.

These first two phases help screen out a vast majority of the drugs that simply don't live up to their promise (in terms of safety and effectiveness).

Some substances that seem to be good treatments in animals can react very differently (or not react at all) in humans. Or there may be problems with negative side effects, minor or major. Or perhaps the dose at which no dangerous side effects occur is too low to be of any therapeutic help. The drugs that survive this gauntlet go on to the final step, Phase III testing.

According to FDA estimates, only one out of every five drugs that are approved for Phase I human trials will make it past Phase III to become standard treatments. The strict tests of safety and effectiveness during Phases I and II are where most of the four out of five drugs that don't make it are eliminated. That means a new drug in a Phase III trial has had most of the bugs worked out of it.

So why do doctors need to do a Phase III trial? They don't always. If there are overwhelmingly positive results from the first two trials, the FDA may approve the drug. But in the vast majority of cases, doctors need more data to confirm safety and effectiveness and to determine conditions of use.

A Phase III trial tests the new drug in greater numbers of people and, on some occasions, for a significantly longer period of time—three or four years, sometimes even longer. Such wider, longer testing helps uncover any long-term side effects, including those that are less common in the general population. It also helps doctors fine-tune how much of the new drug various types of patients should get and how often they should get it over a normal course of treatment.

In some Phase III trials (called "open trials") everybody receives the test substance. In others, the participants are divided into two groups: One group receives the new drug; the other group (control group) gets the best current therapy. If the new drug proves to be overwhelmingly better, the researchers will stop the trial and give the control group the option of getting the new drug.

Nondrug clinical trials in the final stages work the same way: Standard treatment is pitted against a possibly superior treatment. So you just might catch a rising star—a treatment that's already been proven to be as good as the best there is but is on its way to becoming the new standard.

To Test or Not to Test

In general, anyone can try to get into this kind of "final-stage" clinical trial. New drugs, devices, and surgical procedures are being tested for many medical conditions.

But is this approach to treatment really for you?

The people who have the most to gain are those with a disease or disorder for which there is no entirely satisfactory treatment at the present time. But it's a very personal decision: You, with the help of your doctor, have to weigh the risks and the benefits for yourself.

Besides the possibility of getting better-than-the-best treatment, there are some other advantages you might want to consider.

Time ▶ A final-stage clinical trial has one very great benefit: It can offer a promising new treatment much, much sooner than it would normally be available. In the case of a Phase III drug trial, you may get the new treatment five years before it is sold in your local pharmacy.

Quality of Care ▶ Generally, you'll receive more attentive care in a final-stage clinical trial than you would under normal circumstances. (So any idea that you're a guinea pig in these trials is just not true.) The reason for

181

the extra attention is understandable. When your doctor prescribes a proven treatment, he knows what to expect from it. But doctors don't know everything about the experimental treatment. So they need to monitor your health very closely to follow its effects. A trial is, after all, set up to prove that the new treatment is responsible for improvement in your condition.

Anyone entering a clinical trial is given a very thorough physical examination. That's so the physicians can record any health problems you might have that could alter the investigators' interpretation of your response to the new treatment. In scattered cases, doctors have actually discovered life-threatening health problems that the patients were unaware they had before entering the trial! You'll find that the doctors involved in clinical trials are quick to react to any minor health complaint you might develop while in the study. That's so they can record and monitor any side effects of the new treatment. If a patient seems to be having a serious reaction to treatment, that patient is immediately taken out of the trial and treated with standard therapies. And side effects or not, a patient can withdraw from a clinical trial at any time for personal reasons.

Altruism ▶ Participating in a clinical trial has its noble side, too. If the new treatment is beneficial, you've literally assisted in its development and helped everyone else afflicted with the same disease, now and in the future. If the treatment fails to live up to its promise, you've helped further medical knowledge, with little risk to yourself because of all the safeguards built into the testing process. Either way, you can consider yourself something of a medical pioneer.

Getting into a Trial

With three exceptions—AIDS, cancer, and "orphan" (rare) disease trials—there are no hotlines you can call to find out about specific clinical trials. Even if you could have access to the latest medical research, without some medical background you might not be able to fully understand the risks, benefits, or comparative value of various trials. So deciding on a clinical trial is one situation where you absolutely need your physician's guidance.

This doesn't mean you have to be a passive patient. If you have a medical problem for which there are few satisfactory treatments, tell your doctor that you're interested in clinical trials that test standard treatments against new therapies. If your family doctor can't help, ask for the name of a good subspecialist who might. (Pharmaceutical companies often seek out specialists to set up clinical trials of their latest discoveries.)

And any doctor, in private practice or otherwise, can contact medical schools, major medical centers, or the branches of the National Institutes of Health, a federal government agency, to get information about government-sponsored clinical trials.

If you want to do a little preliminary research on your own, here are some leads for you to follow.

■ For information on trials of new cancer treatments, you can contact the National Cancer Institute hotline: (800) 4-CANCER.

■ The AIDS Clinical Trials Information Service can be reached between 9:00 A.M. and 7:00 P.M. eastern time at (800) TRIALS-A.

■ If you have a rare disease or disorder and would like to find more information about it and whether there are any clinical trials under way, contact the National Organization for Rare Disorders at (800) 999-NORD.

Besides these three organizations, you can try calling nonprofit advocacy groups (like the Arthritis Foundation, for example) to see if they can direct you to anyone involved in promising research.

Refer any information you get to your physician, and let him or her help you decide if a particular clinical trial is right for you.

Don't be terribly disappointed if you're unable to find an ongoing trial for your disease. Often it's a matter of timing: A trial starts up and accepts only a certain number of people, getting enough to fill the quota in a few months. It's possible, too, that you might find a trial and

may be too sick—or even too healthy—to be a good subject for certain research.

Questions to Ask

Let's assume that you and your physician have found a final-stage clinical trial that looks promising. You fit

---

ONE PATIENT'S PERSPECTIVE ON BEING IN A CLINICAL TRIAL

When Hank was diagnosed with non-Hodgkin's lymphoma, a cancer of the lymph glands, he was understandably frightened. "I read that my type of cancer had a much poorer survival rate than Hodgkin's disease. I was determined to get the best treatment possible. So I contacted the National Cancer Institute (NCI). They informed me about a clinical trial under way for non-Hodgkin's lymphoma. I was intrigued because I felt that doctors involved in clinical trials are on the cutting edge; this could give me a better shot at a cure. Plus, I liked the idea of contributing to medical knowledge for the benefit of others.

"As it turned out, this particular trial was unusual in that the doctors were testing the possible benefit of beginning treatment at a later stage of the disease. Based on what they knew of this type of cancer, they suspected that up-front treatment, which is the standard protocol, isn't necessary. Patients did just as well—perhaps even better—receiving treatment later on in the disease.

"When I was making the final decision to go on the trial, I asked four of the NCI doctors what they would do if they were in my shoes. They gave me

the patient profile and have a good chance of being accepted. Now what? First, be a smart health consumer: Make sure you understand what the trial will involve. Read over the patient consent form that every clinical trial must provide, then have your doctor look it over. Ask the doctors running the trial to explain anything you don't understand. These consent forms are required to be in plain English—and most actually are very easy to

their personal views—as individuals, not as physicians—about benefits and risks. I decided to participate in the trial, knowing that I might not receive treatment until my disease progressed to a more advanced stage. I was randomly selected for the delayed-treatment group, and I went without treatment for nearly five years after my diagnosis. At that point my cancer-cell type changed and became more aggressive and chemotherapy was begun.

"I never felt like a 'guinea pig' because I had a good idea of what I was getting into. Also, I always felt like the doctors and nurses were giving me the best possible care and being honest with me. They informed me what would happen in each phase of treatment. They told me, for example, that one of the drugs I'd get makes almost everyone nauseated. Sure enough, that was the only drug that made me sick. But it helped that I knew what to expect.

"I've been involved in this trial for ten years now. My disease is currently in remission, but the doctors still check up on me every four or five months. Most of the other patients in the study are also doing well, so it looks like we backed a winner."

read—but you may want clarification on worrisome top-ics, like the risk of negative side effects. Don't be shy about asking!

Once you have a good understanding of what will be done, discuss with your doctor the risks and benefits of the trial in light of the severity of your medical problem. Does the test treatment offer a significantly greater promise of cure, or is it about the same as the standard therapy? The physicians must answer this and similar questions to the satisfaction of the FDA and the Institu-tional Review Board. Make sure you are satisfied with the answers as well. In addition, ask the following questions.

■ How much of my treatment is free under this trial? Many clinical trials offer free treatment. Except under very unusual circumstances, there should be no charge for a test drug. Manufacturers are allowed to recoup some of their costs on new medical devices. Sometimes (depending on who sponsors the trial) there is a charge for the physician's time or other medical supplies. Find out what, if anything, you'll be billed for and if your insurance will cover it.

■ What other costs will be reimbursed? Some trial sponsors pick up the tab for travel expenses and more.

■ Will I have to travel, or can I be treated close to home? Some clinical trials are conducted at only a few medical centers and may require a hospital stay in an-other city. Others can be set up through a local hospital or physician.

It may not make much sense to disrupt your life and get involved with a faraway trial to treat a minor or even serious problem.

Remember, you don't sign your legal rights away when you sign the consent form to participate in a clinical trial. If you feel that the risks of the trial were misrep-resented and you were harmed as a result, you have the right to legal action. Remember, too, that you have the right to drop out of a clinical trial at any point and for any reason.

But if you do join a clinical trial, you have an ethical responsibility to the trial as long as you remain in it. Strict compliance to the treatment regimen not only assures the doctors of accurate results but also assures you of the greatest possible benefits. That way, everybody wins.

The New High-Tech Artery Opener   23

The usual way to get your arteries cleared of plaque (the stuff that obstructs the flow of blood) is like a strange kind of plumbing—widening the drainpipe of a stopped-up sink and leaving behind the sludge that originally clogged it. Doctors, using a procedure called balloon angioplasty, inflate a balloon in the blood vessel, widening its walls so the blood flows freely again. But the debris remains, and so does the potential for another clog. It's an effective and necessary procedure. But the problem is re-stenosis—often plaque obstructs arteries again.

In comes atherectomy, the newest technique for clearing the way through plaque-jammed arteries.

And here's a first: The procedure actually removes the clog. Experts say they don't know for sure yet, but this therapy may become as effective as, and perhaps more effective than, angioplasty and bypass surgery in certain types of artery blockages. Here's what atherectomy can do.

■ Attack plaque in certain vessels where re-stenosis is high

■ Assist in cleaning up residual plaque after angioplasty

■ Offer a less invasive alternative to bypass that gets you in and out of the hospital faster

■ Add an effective treatment, not just for coronary arteries, but also for arteries elsewhere in the body

On the Plaque Attack

How is it done? A motorized device—the size of a wooden match and resembling a miniature drill attached to a long, thin tube—is slipped into the artery through a pencil-sized sheath. (The most widely used of these devices is called the Simpson Atherocath, named after atherectomy pioneer John B. Simpson, M.D.) A spinning, cup-shaped cutter in this "drill" shaves away the plaque that hangs on the vessel walls. These shavings fall into a tiny receptacle near the cutter, which is removed through the sheath, cleaned, and reinserted—most often under local anesthesia without incisions or stitches. The procedure is about as easy on the patient as angioplasty.

Research is encouraging—enough for the Food and Drug Administration to approve the device for this therapy.

In a study, researchers compared 83 atherectomy patients to a similar group who'd chosen angioplasty. For the atherectomy group, the average narrowing of the coronary arteries after the procedure was only 13 percent of the total diameters. The angioplasty group, however, had average narrowings of 37 percent. There was also less incidence of the artery's inner lining being pulled from the vessel—damage that's common with angioplasty.

"The therapy shows special promise for narrowings in the left anterior descending coronary artery [usually the largest coronary artery, which has the highest rate of blockage]," says Jeff Brinker, director of interventional cardiology and associate professor at Johns Hopkins Medical Institutions. "These have high re-stenosis rates—from 25 to 40 percent. Atherectomy may be able to cut that in half."

On the Periphery

Atherectomy is also effective against peripheral vascular disease—clogged arteries in the thighs and legs. At

Johns Hopkins, 53 patients suffering from leg pain (called claudication), nonhealing skin ulcers, or gangrene of the toes had their clogged arteries treated with the Simpson device. The catheter was able to plow through 99 percent of the blocked arteries. After nine months, 86 percent stayed open, with blood flow improving to the extremities 91 percent of the time. These results were similar to what you'd get from angioplasty.

"It's too soon to tell if it'll be more effective than angioplasty in preventing renarrowing of these arteries, but we're optimistic," says Anthony Venbrux, M.D., assistant professor of radiology at Johns Hopkins Hospital and a member of a team of radiologists who perform atherectomies. "We're currently following up on these patients to see." Some benefits were immediate and dramatic—walking improved, ulcers healed, and in some, amputations were prevented.

Atherectomy may be another facet in a tandem attack on arterial plaque. "Atherectomy can be used to improve upon a previous procedure," says Dr. Brinker. "Sometimes after angioplasty, you're left with flaps of tissue that sway against the current of blood in the vessel. And in some cases, when the balloon expands, plaque expands with it and recoils like an elastic band. Atherectomy can be effective in getting rid of the leftover debris."

Even more, atherectomy may save you from surgery. "Having an early surgery can make a later one increasingly difficult," says the researcher. "A less invasive therapy like atherectomy for less severe cases of blockage may allow you to save bypass surgery for a rainy day, if and when you really need it."

Plaque-Mowing Promise

So far, atherectomy shows potential for taking an important place alongside angioplasty in plaque-busting weaponry. But whether atherectomy will surpass angioplasty in effectiveness is unknown. For people suffering from symptoms of clogged arteries, however, atherectomy may offer another choice.

189

This plaque-mower does have one limitation. "The device is difficult to use in smaller vessels," says Dr. Brinker. "But improvements in the catheter may change that."

As the equipment is refined and doctors get more experienced with it, atherectomy's prowess may be greatly enhanced.

Atherectomy for coronary arteries, for now, is available in 50 or 60 institutions across the country. Among them are Johns Hopkins Medical Institutions in Baltimore, Sequoia Hospital in northern California, the Mayo Clinic in Rochester, Minnesota, Beth Israel Hospital in Boston, and the University of Michigan. For treatment of peripheral vascular disease, the technique is available at many medical centers in this country.

For information on the procedure, you can call Johns Hopkins at (301) 955-5687 for peripheral vascular disease and (301) 955-6086 for coronary artery disease.

24   Update on Psoriasis

Psoriasis sufferers, take heart—not the proverbial heartbreak. While it's true that the disorder's behavior is capricious and unpredictable, you may not have to suffer this interminable, sometimes itchy, unsightly skin condition any longer. The frequency and severity of psoriasis flare-ups can be lessened, doctors tell us. First, you have to learn to recognize and minimize the "triggering factors." And, in the event of a flare-up, talk with your doctor about how you might benefit from one of the latest medical treatments.

While you may have to experiment a bit, "Everybody can be helped, depending on how much time and effort they're willing to put into it," says Cynthia Guzzo, M.D., director of the University of Pennsylvania's Psoriasis Clinic.

Psoriasis is skin growth gone awry. Normally, skin cells mature and shed in 28 to 30 days, making way for new cells. In psoriasis, new skin cells develop seven times faster than normal. Poorly developed psoriatic skin cells can't shed fast enough to keep pace with the rapid growth. Instead, they pile up, forming raised, scaly plaques. The layers closest to the body surface appear red because the affected area is inflamed. As the dead cells are pushed farther from the skin surface, they form silvery white scales over the plaques. Generally, these scaly, red, telltale signs of psoriasis show up on the elbows, knees, scalp, and lower back, but other parts of the body can be involved.

Snuff Out the Spark

Experts are still looking for the actual cause of psoriasis. They know it's not contagious and think there may be a genetic link. In one out of three cases, the disorder can be traced through the family, although it sometimes skips a generation.

But having the tendency simply sets the stage for a flare-up. People with the disorder can go through periods during which their skin looks normal. That's because psoriasis itself is like a bomb—something must trigger its fuse to set off an explosion. Unfortunately, that something could be just about anything. Experts have pinpointed some key triggers, among them possibly the climate, damage to the skin (from dryness, to a scratch, to sunburn, to chafing clothing, for example), a reaction to certain drugs, and infections (such as strep throat). Recently a clear link has been made between stress and psoriasis.

To prevent psoriasis attacks and minimize their severity, try to heed the following advice.

Moisturize ▶ Skin that's prone to psoriasis tends to be dry. Lubricating is particularly important during the winter months, a time when psoriasis tends to flare up because of the dry, cold air.

191

Avoid bathing with perfumed and deodorant soaps, which can be drying. A 5- to 10-minute bath in comfortably warm water with a superfatted cleansing bar is your best bet. Just be sure to rinse well; soap residue can be irritating and drying. Then, while your skin is still damp, seal in the moisture with petrolatum, lanolin, or any good over-the-counter moisturizer. Perfumed or tinted brands are okay if you're not allergic to them. (Psoriasis and skin allergies don't necessarily go hand in hand.) Running a humidifier, especially during drier weather, is also recommended.

Avoid Prolonged Sun Exposure ▶ Sunburn, like other skin irritations, can worsen a psoriasis outbreak. "Most people know their skin type and can tell how much they can get before they start to burn," says Christopher E. M. Griffiths, M.D., an assistant professor of dermatology at the University of Michigan Medical School, Ann Arbor, but he recommends you consult a dermatologist anyway to determine a safe length of exposure and appropriate sunscreen, which should be used all over.

Limit Your Alcohol Intake ▶ There appears to be something to the alcohol/psoriasis connection. In a Finnish study, doctors noted a higher level of alcohol consumption among patients with severe psoriasis. Among a control group of 285 patients with other skin problems (such as dermatitis and acne), alcohol consumption was much lower. What's more, one in three of the psoriasis patients reported that drinking seemed to worsen their condition, whereas only one in nine of the controls reported such a connection with their skin problem.

Doctors aren't sure whether it's the alcohol or the stress (which leads some people to drink) that exacerbates psoriasis symptoms—or rather that worsening symptoms prompt many to turn to the bottle.

Other research suggests that alcohol increases the activity of a certain kind of white blood cell in psoriasis patients, but not in people who don't have the disease. This increase was most evident in patients who said that drinking made their psoriasis worse. Thus the researchers theorized a connection between the alcohol-induced activity of white blood cells and worsening of the patients' psoriasis.

Don't Get Irritated (Literally) ▶ Psoriasis often flares up in areas traumatized by a scratch, bump, or abrasion. While it's not always possible to protect your body from such assaults, you can avoid snug-fitting or elasticized clothing. Bra straps and tight waistbands rubbing on the skin are often culprits in a localized flare-up, says Dr. Griffiths.

Beware of Certain Medications ▶ A few drugs have been identified as occasionally causing psoriasis flare-ups. These include antimalarials, propranolol hydrochloride and other beta-blocker medications to control high blood pressure, lithium, the heart medication quinidine gluconate, and topical, or rub-on, steroids (when used for prolonged periods). Talk with your doctor or pharmacist if you suspect your medication may be getting under your skin.

Don't Get Irritated Emotionally ▶ Research substantiates a connection between stress and psoriasis. "We've explained in the lab how factors produced by nerve fibers in the skin are linked to the earliest phases of inflammation," says George F. Murphy, M.D., professor of dermatology and pathology at the University of Pennsylvania, who studies skin abnormalities. In a complicated process, nerves cause the inner lining of the blood vessels to stick to white blood cells, which normally travel freely throughout the body. The white blood cells then pass through the walls of the blood vessels into the tissue and cause inflammation. "If we accept this mind/body link, we can think about using stress management to attack the inflammation cascade of events very early, perhaps even before it happens," he adds.

Stress management can be as simple as time management, says Iona Ginsburg, M.D., a New York psychiatrist who counsels psoriasis patients. "It makes you feel more competent to handle your responsibilities, decreases your tension, and allows you more time to take care of your skin. You have a sense of taking charge, so you feel more in control of this troublesome problem," she says.

Several experts interviewed say popular relaxation techniques are excellent ways of defusing stress before it aggravates your psoriasis. And John Koo, M.D., a dermatologist and psychiatrist at the Psoriasis Treatment Center at the University of California, San Francisco, says many of his patients show more rapid and sustained improvement when they get psychological counseling to address personal problems that are causing them undue stress.

Look After Your Overall Physical State ▶ "The skin is like any other organ of the body—it's going to be influenced by a good, balanced diet and adequate exercise," says David L. Cram, M.D., a clinical professor of dermatology at the University of California, San Francisco. Other experts interviewed concur.

Extinguishing Flare-Ups

Despite all these precautions, you may still suffer an occasional flare-up. If you do, you'll need to see your physician. Left untended, psoriasis usually doesn't go away. But with appropriate treatment, psoriasis can go into remission for months, years, possibly even for the rest of your life.

What the doctor recommends depends on the extent of your psoriasis and your response to medications. "The treatment really has to be tailored to the individual patient," says Elizabeth Knobler, M.D., director of the psoriasis and phototherapy treatment center at New York's Columbia–Presbyterian Medical Center.

The preventive measures mentioned above are also useful in minimizing the severity of a flare-up, but it's likely that you'll need at least one of the following medically approved medications to extinguish the flame.

Steroid Creams ▶ These are also known as corticoids, cortisones, or corticosteroids. Applied daily to limited areas, these creams help reduce inflammation. They are generally recommended for short-term treatment; prolonged use can actually damage the skin and exacerbate the condition.

Coal Tar ▶ This is an old-time remedy that reduces inflammation, itching, and scaling. Now available in bath and shampoo formulas, as well as in rub-on ointments and creams, some of today's products don't have the objectionable color or smell of the original. Some of these are OTCs; some are prescription drugs. They're often used on patients who develop resistance to or have side effects from steroids.

PUVA ▶ "P" refers to the medication, psoralen; "UVA" refers to ultraviolet light, a component of natural sunlight. While it's true that sunburn can worsen psoriasis, a controlled dose of UVA (administered in the doctor's office along with a pill containing psoralen, a light-sensitizing drug) can actually have a healing effect. The therapy entails about three treatments a week; exposure is gradually increased to avoid burning. Usually, the skin returns to normal within 20 to 30 treatments. PUVA has proved to be very effective in at least 80 percent of cases. But be aware that this treatment carries all the negative side effects associated with sun exposure—that is, premature skin aging, as well as increased risk of skin cancer and cataracts.

Anthralin ▶ This also comes in preparations for both the body and the scalp. Formerly, this treatment had to be administered in a hospital or doctor's office because of its potential to irritate normal skin and permanently stain anything it came in contact with. New formulations of the medication, however, have been introduced that significantly reduce these hazards.

Etretinate (Tegison) ▶ This is a vitamin A derivative, much like Accutane (which has been used to combat acne). The drug is taken orally once a day. Warning: Like its cousin Accutane, etretinate can cause birth defects; don't risk it if you are pregnant. It may also contribute to bone calluses and spurs, dry and fragile skin, and high blood cholesterol, so doctors avoid long-term use.

Methotrexate ▶ Doctors reserve this for very severe psoriasis cases that resist all other treatment. Used primarily as an anticancer agent, this drug is potentially toxic to the liver; patients must have liver biopsies at intervals during treatment. The drug is taken orally once a week.

More Help on the Way

Fortunately, your options are expanding. Here are several promising experimental medications.

Vitamin D ▶ An active form of vitamin D—1,25-dihydroxyvitamin D—has demonstrated exciting potential. Used topically or orally, it appears to stop skin cells from growing wildly and makes them mature normally.

Michael F. Holick, M.D., Ph.D., director of the vitamin D laboratory at Boston City Hospital, who has been studying the vitamin derivative, says 90 percent of his patients showed a marked decrease in scales and a clearing up of inflammation within two to four weeks when they applied a topical form of D once a day. Sixty-five percent of the patients who took it orally once a day showed similar improvement in two to three months. Unlike current medications, active D seems to have fewer side effects. None of the problems associated with the vitamin have turned up in the studies so far. However, psoriasis returns when the treatment is stopped.

This medication may already be in use in Europe, says Dr. Holick, and he's hopeful that it will be approved for use in the United States within the next few years. Standard vitamin D supplements are not effective, he adds, and can cause toxicity if taken in high doses.

Fish Oil ▶ This has shown some promise as an adjunct to current treatments (used alone, its effects are minimal). In a 12-week study at the Skin Research Foundation of California in Santa Monica, 24 psoriasis patients who were being treated with Acitretin were given six 1-gram capsules of fish oil as a daily supplement. All showed more improvement in their condition than a control group that was taking Acitretin alone. Also, the fish oil seems to counter one of the adverse effects of the drug by lowering the levels of certain fats in the blood that the medication tends to raise.

Nicholas J. Lowe, M.D., director of the foundation, says other studies have shown fish oil enhances the effects of light therapy. The omega-3 fatty acids found in the oil are known to reduce the levels of other acids in the body that cause inflammation, including that associated with psoriasis.

Until more research is done, it wouldn't hurt to simply eat more fish high in omega-3's, such as herring, mackerel, and salmon, says Dr. Lowe. It may help keep *your* skin scales to a minimum.

Acitretin ▶ Like etretinate, this vitamin A derivative can clear severe psoriasis symptoms when taken orally once a day. But, even better, it is eliminated a lot more quickly from the body, so the side effects, such as high blood cholesterol and bone spurs, may be more manageable and reversible. It may also be safer to use in fertile women than etretinate (provided they avoid pregnancy while taking it and for two months after taking it). It's now awaiting approval by the Food and Drug Administration.

For more information, contact the National Psoriasis Foundation, which many of the experts interviewed recommended as a terrific source of information and support: NPF, Suite 210, 6443 SW Beaverton Highway, Portland, OR 97221.

197

Everyday
Health
Concerns

Deep-Down, Dog-Tired? 25

Your spouse says it's all in your head. You say it's in your head, your neck, your arms, your legs. You're tired down to your toes, and you're tired all the time—just like up to 20 to 30 percent of people in America who walk into their doctor's office. But your doctor says it's not chronic fatigue syndrome—that diagnosis requires plenty of symptoms above and beyond fatigue. And he's ruled out many of the usual instigators of fatigue like hypothyroidism, not putting in enough sleep time, anemia, and anxiety disorder. So what is causing you to feel like you're walking under water, five miles down?

Maybe something right out of left field—like one of the seven unexpected causes of chronic fatigue we cover here. The experts interviewed say that these factors are capable of draining your energy, yet can be overlooked, even by physicians. If you've been feeling fatigue for months and don't have anything to pin it on, be sure to see a doctor. The problem could be simple or complex. And it could be one of the "mysterious seven," which means there are ways to put the energy drain in reverse.

Moving and Shaking

You sit behind a desk all day and you never overexert yourself. Still, you're always tired. How can that be? Maybe your problem is a lack of exertion.

There's not a lot of research that shows that not exercising makes you lazy. But it's a logical conclusion most experts have come to—that not being active creates a pattern of inactivity, lethargy, and fatigue. "It's common sense," says D. W. Edington, Ph.D., director of the Fitness Research Center at the University of Michigan. "The body at rest tends to remain at rest."

On the other hand, regular physical conditioning results in greater overall energy. So someone who works out regularly probably feels much more energetic throughout the day than a couch potato.

But besides keeping your energy up on a long-term basis, exercise can energize you on the spot. And the effects can keep you going for up to 2 hours, says Robert Thayer, Ph.D., a California State University psychology professor.

In early studies he conducted, Dr. Thayer showed that moderate exercise enhances energy better than inactivity, suggesting that walking could make you feel a lot more "rested" than would resting itself. And most recently, in a study of 18 volunteers, Dr. Thayer compared the effects of taking a 10-minute walk and eating a candy bar on the subjects' energy and tension.

He found that walking was associated with higher energy and lower tension than was snacking, with exercise's effects lasting up to 2 hours. Even after 1 hour, the walkers had more energy and were less tense than before they started walking. Snacking, of course, did boost energy. But after an hour, it caused increased tiredness and more tension than walking. And subjects were actually more tense and tired than before they ate the candy bar.

That's important to know if you need a quick pick-me-up before an important meeting or a busy afternoon. "The usual way that people act in that regard is to have a quick cup of coffee or some quick sugar snack," says Dr. Thayer. "The walk is clearly more useful than either of those things."

Exercise also improves the quality of your sleep, which could in itself reduce fatigue. Ask Robert Sweetgall, president of Creative Walking, Inc., who took a cross-country walk—11,208 miles, through 50 states, in 52 weeks. He averaged only 5 hours of sleep a night after averaging 31 miles of walking a day.

"Think about the days you're outdoors hiking, gardening, or walking, and how you sleep those nights," he says. "Then think about the days when you're cooped up in the office sitting on your rear at 1 calorie a minute.

You don't need to be a rocket scientist to figure out that you sleep best on the days when you burn more calories."

So here's some advice if you want to start fighting fatigue with regular workouts.

See a Doctor First ▶ If your fatigue is due to some medical problem, exercise may worsen your symptoms. So it's important to rule out any medical disorders with your doctor before embarking on a serious exercise program.

Choose Your Workout Well ▶ Keep in mind that vigorous exercise can initially wear you out. After doing vigorous aerobic exercise for about 30 minutes, you'll feel fatigued. It will take about an hour after your workout before you experience the energy-enhancing effects. But a less intensive workout—like a brisk walk—can give you the energizing effect much sooner. Even during the walk you may start to get a "lift."

Ease into It ▶ The "no pain, no gain" theory has no place with beginners, especially those who are already pained by fatigue. If you have any pain—either while you're exercising or the next day—you're probably doing too much. Take your exercise program slowly and advance gradually, says Dr. Thayer. But most important, stick to it.

Set aside 30 minutes several times a week to do moderate exercise, like walking. As a guide, try the "talk test." If you can't talk comfortably while you're walking, you're probably pushing yourself too hard. And, of course, if you experience any chest pains or dizziness, it's time to get off the track and into the hospital.

Beware of Late-Night Workouts ▶ If exercise will pick you up when you're down, that's not what you want at bedtime. While some people can work out at any hour and still get plenty of sleep, others need to stop vigorous exercise a few hours before going to bed—or face hours of tossing and turning and, no doubt, tomorrow's fatigue.

Rest Assured

You're early to bed, early to rise—and still you're exhausted all the time. Why?

One often-undetected cause of fatigue is obstructive sleep apnea (OSA). Most common among middle-aged men, OSA is the most prevalent kind of sleep apnea, accounting for about 90 percent of all cases. It occurs when breathing is blocked by closure of the throat tissues—you actually stop breathing for 20 to 40 seconds at a time while you're asleep.

When this happens, you're forced to wake up to breathe again, although the next day you don't remember the interruption in your sleep. The awakening is brief, but it can happen hundreds of times a night, so you lose a substantial amount of sleep. And because deep sleep is disturbed, you also miss out on the most important sleep—the restorative time—allowing unrelenting fatigue to set in.

But fatigue isn't the only problem OSA can create. Doctors suspect that 2,000 to 3,000 people die in their sleep every year from causes related to obstructive sleep apnea. Excessive sleepiness is the second-highest cause of driving fatalities, and the risk is particularly high for OSA sufferers. And OSA is linked to heart disease and high blood pressure. That has to do with the fact that in OSA the intake of oxygen is reduced during sleep. Reduced oxygen levels can lead to slowed heart rate and abnormal heart rhythms—even heart attack. While you may not realize you have sleep apnea, your spouse probably will. It's characterized by loud snoring along with stoppages in breathing (although not all snorers have apnea). You may notice a morning headache upon awakening.

If you think sleep apnea could be at the root of your fatigue, see a doctor right away. As soon as possible, you need to be evaluated by a physician who specializes in sleep disorders and who will suggest an all-night sleep recording to get a diagnosis. (Such recordings may also be used to monitor treatment.)

Many of these sleep experts are at sleep disorders centers. There are an estimated 1,000 such centers in the country where you can go to determine if your sleep is what's making you sleepy. For more information on sleep disorders and on the centers near you, write to the American Sleep Disorders Association, 604 Second Street SW, Rochester, MN 55902.

If it's determined that you have sleep apnea, there's plenty of treatment available to you. One option is drugs that stimulate respiration. Another is surgery. For many OSA sufferers, the most effective means is the use of a nasal continuous positive airway pressure (nasal CPAP) during sleep. The nasal CPAP, a nonsurgical treatment, is a mask that fits over the nose and uses a pump to generate air pressure and prevent the airways from being obstructed.

Lifestyle changes may also help you reduce or eliminate OSA. Here are the two most effective steps.

Cut the Fat ▶ Losing weight can be helpful—possibly because extra tissue in the neck and throat, combined with poor muscle tone, restricts the upper airway, making your chances of obstruction greater. Studies have shown that a weight loss of 10 to 25 percent can eliminate OSA or reduce the number of episodes.

Ban the Booze ▶ Skipping alcohol can also reduce the severity of OSA. Since alcohol works as a depressant in the central nervous system, it increases muscle relaxation and so enhances airway blockage. (Too much alcohol near bedtime can also interfere with the quality of your sleep, inducing fatigue.)

Tossing and Turning

About 8 percent of Americans—and at least 15 percent of those over 50—experience what doctors call "periodic leg movements" during the night. And many people aren't even aware that they have the problem. The movements vary among individuals, normally involving a motion in one leg. But they can mean anything from a toe-flex to a full-fledged kick that's sure to catch a bed partner's attention.

Sleep disorder experts aren't exactly sure what causes these involuntary movements—technically, nocturnal myoclonus. Some suspect lower back injuries to be a cause, while others suspect central nervous system problems. What they do know is that these movements can cause fatigue. That's because they can occur hundreds of times a night; they might disappear for an hour, then return to occur every 20 or 30 seconds. And since they can interrupt your sleep in the process, the result can be fatigue.

Periodic leg movements are different from hypnic jerks—the classic "falling dreams" that jerk you awake just when you're falling asleep. They're also different from, but related to, restless-leg syndrome, which involves a deep discomfort in the limbs.

People with restless-leg syndrome describe it as a creepy sensation that's alleviated only by rubbing, shaking, or moving your legs. But relief is only temporary; soon you have to move again.

Those with restless-leg syndrome probably realize they have a problem—they have a hard time falling asleep because of their need to move around. But you might have periodic leg movements when you're asleep and not even realize your sleep is being disturbed every so often—up to 400 times a night.

If you have periodic movements, your main cue is sleepiness during the day. You'll probably hear complaints from your bed partner about your kicking during the night. Less common is a feeling of muscular fatigue in your legs in the morning, as if you've been running a marathon in the night.

If you think your legs are doing laps throughout the night, visit a sleep disorders center. Periodic leg movements probably can't be eliminated completely, but medication can help reduce the number of arousal episodes during the night. And that could reduce your fatigue.

Breathe Easy

Another common, often-overlooked cause of fatigue is simply breathing wrong. As many as 25 to 40 percent of patients who seek medical help for any reason are said to have chronic hyperventilation syndrome (HVS), which results from poor breathing patterns.

HVS patients breathe shallowly and rapidly, leading to hyperventilation—the excessive loss of carbon dioxide. Hyperventilation causes fatigue because the loss of carbon dioxide affects the blood's hemoglobin, making it less able to carry oxygen throughout the body. So even though you're breathing quickly, you're getting less air.

You may not realize it if you have HVS. Most HVS patients think they just can't catch their breath and assume they have a breathing problem, but rarely recognize it as hyperventilation. Besides inability to catch your breath, look for clues like anxiety, plus tingling, coldness, or numbness in the fingers. Some people with HVS yawn or sigh frequently. That's because they hold their breath to make up for the carbon dioxide lost in hyperventilating.

HVS can be caused by many medical disorders—among them, heart and kidney disease, anemia, diabetes, and hypertension. Stress is a big cause of HVS because it leads you to tense your muscles—not only the ones in your neck but also those in your diaphragm. The result is that your diaphragm can't move freely, and you compensate by breathing more quickly.

Oddly enough, some develop HVS from simple good posture, says Robert Fried, Ph.D., of the Institute for Rational Emotive Therapy in New York City, who is author of *The Breath Connection* and *The Hyperventilation Syndrome*. By keeping your tummy firmly tucked in when you stand up straight, you may be tensing the diaphragm muscles and limiting their movement during breathing. So try not to tense your muscles all the time.

Examining the movement of your diaphragm is one way to tell if you're not breathing correctly. From a sitting or standing position, put one hand on your chest, one hand on your abdomen. Then watch your hands as you breathe. If they don't rise with each breath, you may be taking rapid, shallow breaths and hyperventilating.

According to Dr. Fried, most family doctors don't readily recognize HVS. So if you suspect your breathing is what's got you dragging, read up on hyperventilation and direct your doctor's attention to it. If he thinks you're a candidate for HVS, you may want to see a specialist who can literally teach you to breathe again. Dr. Fried uses a breathing biofeedback system to show his patients a computer analysis of their breathing patterns and where they're going wrong.

Most people can "relearn" breathing techniques. But some have trouble. For them the simplest treatment for HVS is to just keep their mouth closed. If you breathe from your nose, you can't hyperventilate—the nasal passages are too narrow, says Dr. Fried. By doing so, you could do more than breathe a little easier; you just might get your energy back in the long run.

Fatiguing Feelings

Another medical problem associated with fatigue is depression. By depression, doctors don't just mean the blues. But real depression—major depressive disorder—is classified as lasting at least two weeks and impairing your ability to function at home or at work.

It's also associated with major changes in the body. According to the American Psychiatric Association's criteria for diagnosing depression, symptoms include loss of interest or pleasure in all or almost all usual activities, poor appetite, feelings of worthlessness, and—you guessed it—fatigue.

Depression has a great effect on sleep, which further complicates the problem of fatigue. Some people with depression have insomnia, while others sleep all the time. Depression is also known to cause significant fatigue. And doctors agree that treating the depression should help alleviate the fatigue.

Most cases of depression are treated by a family doctor, says Susan Abbey, M.D., who specializes in psychiatry for the medically ill at Toronto General Hospital. But often your doctor will refer you to a psychiatrist for assessment.

Treatment varies according to the patient. Some do better on antidepressant medications. You should reap the full benefits of antidepressant medication within four to six weeks. But the symptoms begin disappearing step by step, in different phases, says Dr. Abbey.

Other patients prefer cognitive therapy—examining their thought patterns and replacing negative thoughts with positive ones.

We've already said exercise can help reduce feelings of fatigue, but it can give a lift to your mood, too. In a study of 45 college students at the University of Kansas, researchers demonstrated the antidepressive effects of exercise. The students were all under high stress and had reported a number of negative life events during the previous year. None of them exercised.

They were then placed in three groups—one that exercised for 11 weeks, another that practiced relaxation techniques, and one that did no exercise or relaxation training.

The study showed that those in the exercise group showed greater reductions in self-reported depression scores by a midpoint in the exercise program than students in both other groups. And those who were the most depressed before the exercise program showed the most improvement.

Not Enough Stress

Sure, you know stress can make you feel fatigued. But did you know that a lack of stress can contribute to fatigue?

Some say there's a delicate balance to be maintained between boredom and burnout. Long ago two researchers proposed that each person has an optimal point of stress. Their theory holds that as stress increases, so does performance—to a point. If you're stressed past the point of your optimal performance, your performance dips. On the other hand, if you don't have enough stress, you aren't motivated to perform at all.

"It's sort of like the tension on a violin string," explains Paul J. Rosch, M.D., president of the American Institute of Stress. "If you have too much tension, the string is going to break. If you don't have enough tension, it's not going to make any music."

No matter what job you have, you may find yourself feeling understressed and therefore fatigued, says Dennis T. Jaffe, Ph.D., author of *Take This Job and Love It*. This happens "by not pushing through to continually develop your skills and abilities, by trying to coast by on what you know instead of trying to expand and enrich and grow."

So how do you get going when you have no get-up-and-go?

Restress ▶ "You have to find out what works for you," says Dr. Rosch. "Some people leave everything to the last minute so they can get that little surge of adrenaline. Or they have to get to the airport just at the last minute."

Since a lack of creative engagement is taxing, says Dr. Jaffe, you should try getting involved in more things, like learning a new skill or becoming part of a group of active, committed people.

Help Someone Else ▶ "I used to write prescriptions for becoming a volunteer," says John Renner, M.D., a consumer health expert at the Consumer Health Information Research Institute in Kansas City, Missouri. "I recommend that you get into something where you are needed. Work with children, work with senior citizens, work with an agency that needs your help." That interest in others' lives—and extra activity in your own—just might lift you out of understress.

Cutting Calories

When your calorie intake dips too low—because you're dieting or are too rushed to eat correctly—fatigue can hit you hard. It hits so hard because you're not taking in enough calories to sustain your body's normal functions.

In normal weight loss, you expend more calories than you take in. So your body turns to its reserves and burns its "stored" calories—your fat deposits. But when your calorie intake is restricted too much, your body itself starts to function poorly. "The body starts to live off itself," says *Prevention* adviser Manfred Kroger, Ph.D., professor of food science at Pennsylvania State University. "This whole process is abnormal and very stressful to the body, and one of the many symptoms of this type of stress is fatigue."

So to avoid fatigue caused by a restricted diet, don't cut your calorie intake below 1,000 a day. (Most good weight-loss plans set caloric minimums even higher than this.) Plus, exercise can add an additional 1,000 calories to your body's requirements.

Diets that would bar you from eating a variety of foods may be as bad as those that drastically restrict your calories. They may put you at risk for below-normal nutrient intakes or even nutrient deficiency.

So here's what to do in order to lose weight without losing energy.

Forgo the Fat ▶ Fat calories are more easily turned into body fat than either protein or carbohydrate calories are. Plus, fats contain more calories per gram of food than the other two. So replacing fatty foods with high-carbohydrate foods like fruits, vegetables, grains, and pasta can give you an edge in losing weight—without drastically restricting calories. In fact, most weight-loss

209

experts recommend that people count grams of fat, not calories, to shed pounds. A diet containing less than 30 percent of its calories from fat can help most people lose weight and lower disease risk factors.

Lose in Moderation ▶ It's reasonable to lose 1 or 2 pounds a week. Any more than that is getting risky. Drastic weight loss increases your chances of fatigue and gallstone formation. It also can lead to heart problems, says Steven Heymsfield, M.D., director of the Weight Control Unit at St. Luke's Obesity Research Center in New York City.

26 8 Tips for Sneeze-Free Walking

Late summer and early fall promise those of us with weed-pollen and mold-related allergies a wicked bout with stuffy noses and itchy eyes.

In general, seasonal allergy (hay fever) sufferers can expect to experience the most discomfort from August through October. That's when big offenders, such as ragweed, pigweed, and lamb's-quarters, pollinate over most of the country. In August, mold allergies can also be especially troublesome, since mold spore levels, spurred by summer rains, tend to peak.

If you're an allergy-ridden walker, this can turn a pleasant outdoor stroll into a nose-blowing, sniffling, red-eyed ordeal. What can you do besides give up walking 'til the first frost?

Identify Your Personal Allergens ▶ An allergist can perform skin tests to determine exactly what allergens are triggering your symptoms. Knowing the specific offenders can help you plan your walking program in order to avoid them.

If you're allergic to weed pollen, for example, you'll

be more comfortable if you take your walk later in the day, because weeds typically release their pollen early in the morning.

If you're allergic to molds, you'll do better by walking immediately after a rain. You'll have a few hours' lag time between the time the rain wets everything and the time molds start producing spores like crazy.

Premedicate ▶ Taking over-the-counter (OTC) antihistamines may help you keep walking through the allergy season. Your pharmacist or doctor can help you choose the one that's right for you. Antihistamines are preventive medications. So for maximum effectiveness, you can schedule your walk ½ hour after taking your medication.

Some antihistamines can cause drowsiness or a jittery feeling. These side effects can sometimes be lessened by starting with one-quarter to one-half of the recommended dosage and increasing your intake daily, working up to a full dose over a period of three or four days. If OTC medications don't do the trick, you might want to ask your doctor about prescription antihistamines. The prescription drugs are available in several forms, including pills, eyedrops that relieve itching eyes, and nasal sprays that prevent allergy-caused stuffy noses.

Try Allergy Shots ▶ These must be taken all year long in order for them to be effective during the allergy season. If medication doesn't bring you relief, talk to an allergist about this option for next year.

Get Rid of Excess Pollen ▶ If you shower and wash your hair after you walk, you can rinse away most of the pollen you picked up. If you can't fit a shower into your schedule, try washing your hands and face and rinsing your eyes to remove any pollen.

Don a Surgical Mask ▶ If your symptoms are really annoying, you may not mind looking like Dr. Kildare. A mask offers some protection by filtering pollen. Look for the ones designed to protect industrial workers and home

211
■

renovators. They're available in hardware stores and home centers.

Stretch Indoors ▶ If you like to do stretching exercises before you walk, do them indoors rather than outside so your exposure to allergens is less. Your body reacts cumulatively, so the less exposure to pollen or mold, the less severe your reaction.

Steer Clear of Vacant Lots ▶ Offending weeds tend to proliferate in vacant lots, or any area that is not mown regularly. To avoid them, you may have to find another route.

Check the Pollen Count ▶ Daily readings on pollen and mold levels are often included in newspaper, radio, or television weather forecasts. If it's going to be a very bad day (on windy days, for example, pollen is really flying), consider an indoor treadmill workout or head for a mall, where you can walk in climate-controlled, pollen-free comfort.

SEEKING SNEEZE-FREE WALKING TRIPS

If you're planning a walking vacation and you have allergies, be sure to take your schnozzola into consideration. To find out if your particular allergy culprits will be in bloom when you arrive at your destination, call the Asthma and Allergy Foundation of America's allergy hotline at (800) 7-ASTHMA. Tell them where and when you plan to travel, and they'll tell you what allergens are particular hazards for that location and time of year. For more extensive information on seasonal allergies throughout the country, send a self-addressed stamped envelope to the foundation at 1717 Massachusetts Avenue NW, Suite 305, Washington, DC 20036.

Stretches for   27
Stressed-Out Muscles

By Charles Norelli, M.D.

My medical specialty is one few people know about. As a physiatrist (fizz-ee-A-trist), I deal chiefly with rehabilitating injured patients. But as a doctor who also treats a wide spectrum of physical problems, I see many people who are suffering from chronic, debilitating pain caused by everything from old injuries to poor posture and hyperstress.

With this medical background, I couldn't help noticing that certain yoga postures—stretches, actually—focus on the very same muscles that cause so much trouble for my patients. Maybe whoever came up with yoga centuries ago had fibromyalgia—a syndrome of multiple areas of tenderness, often relieved by gentle muscle stretching. There has to be a reason why yoga has survived so long—longer, perhaps than any other technique.

Anyway, physiatrists specialize in the stuff that accounts for about 40 percent of us—our muscles. You're probably familiar with superficial surface muscles like the pectorals, abdominals, and biceps that give bodybuilders their dramatic, armor-plated look. But I'm more concerned with lesser-known muscles that lie deep beneath the surface and have names that sound like prehistoric animals, such as the quadratus lumborum (under the spine) and the psoas major (running from groin to spine).

When some of the fibers in these muscles get tense, tight, shortened, overworked, strained, or weakened, they can develop "trigger points" that telegraph pain to other parts of the body. Often the origin of the problem is hidden. Headaches, numbness in the hand, or sciatica-like stabbing pain all suggest other origins—nerve problems, for instance. But the underlying cause (and I mean that literally) is often abused muscles.

Puzzling pain needs to be evaluated medically before any treatment is begun. And many of the people I see (excluding accident victims) have been to other specialists who, not finding any obvious cause for the pain, refer them to our hospital. By observing the patient's posture, inquiring about his or her habits, and examining and feeling the body for tender areas, I can often ferret out the hidden trouble and guide the patient through stretches that return them to wellness.

As a Western physician who is admittedly no expert in yoga, I have freely adapted the ancient art to my own purposes and style. The postures that follow employ only the physical, and not the mental or spiritual aspects, of yoga (which are no doubt very valuable). For convenience, none of them need be done on the floor, as real yoga is. They can all be done in your office, in fact. Think of these stretches as both a preventive routine (for deterring stressed-out muscles) and a broad-spectrum muscle-soothing therapy for a range of common symptoms stemming from modern lifestyles.

Do them slowly, gently, and with concentration on proper form. Don't hold your breath; breathe regularly. Only one to three repetitions of each posture need be done—you can get through the whole routine in a few minutes. But those few minutes can be very valuable. The kinds of problems we're attacking, like constant tension and poor posture, tend to be self-perpetuating unless the cycle is broken.

Ear-to-Knee Stretch

I'll start with the most valuable stretch, because it relaxes the quadratus lumborum, in my view the most overlooked source of low back pain. The quadratus lies deep beneath the spinal muscles and joins the pelvis to the twelfth rib. When tight or tender, it can pull you down, or off to one side, causing you to shuffle. Or there may be unrelenting pain at the belt level in your low back. Sound familiar? The causes of a whacked-out quadratus are legion. A common one is prolonged sitting, es-

214
■

pecially if you have a habit of leaning to one side, as you might do when watching TV or talking on the phone. Awkward lifting, sustained overload from gardening, or scrubbing the floor can also do it. So can a fall. Or even a quick stooping movement when your torso is twisted. The quadratus is also irritated by poor posture, scoliosis, or having one leg shorter than the other. The ear-to-knee stretch helps relax this troublesome muscle.

Sitting in a chair, spread your legs apart, place your palms on your ankles, and let your torso sink between your knees to loosen your back a bit. Then slowly bend your torso to the left, until your left ear touches your left knee. Rotate your head slowly to the right. If you are so tight you can't comfortably reach this position, come as close as you can without causing strain. Now slowly raise your right arm until it is just sort of hanging over your head. Hold this for 10 seconds, then slowly raise your torso. Repeat on the opposite side, with your right ear to your right knee.

Wave to the Sun

Another muscle—a pair, actually—that you probably never heard of is the psoas (*SO-as*) minor and major, or the "tenderloin" muscles. They are quite long, extending from the thighs and hip joint right up to the lower spine. They can both tighten up from too much sitting (a nearly universal problem these days), causing pain in the middle of the back.

To stretch them, we do a version of part of the Sun Salutation series of postures, which every yoga student knows.

Stand with your feet together and your toes pointed directly ahead. Bring your left foot backward and your right foot forward, taking care to keep your toes pointed straight ahead. Raise your left arm straight overhead; keep your right arm at your side. Now bend your knees slightly and tip your torso back somewhat. You should feel a good, gentle stretch under your belt on the left side. Breathing regularly (as always in these postures), hold for 10 seconds or so, and return. Repeat on the other side. This is a good stretch you can do before and after those long meetings or a major bout of reading.

Neck Looseners

I once had a patient who complained of chronic neck pain. She blamed it on having to tilt her head out of the water to breathe while swimming laps. When I pestered her for more details about her life, she thought a bit and mentioned that, oh, yes, she played violin for 3 hours every day. Aha!

The point is, know thyself. Those recurring headaches could persist because you sit at a desk all day with your head tilted down toward a computer screen. Also, in winter, we tend to try to contract our neck, turtlelike, to keep warm.

A series of neck stretches, culled from yogic neck rolls, can help loosen three different and important muscle groups.

The splenii (*SPLEE-nee-eye*) are the muscles that run up the back of your neck on both sides of your spine. Keeping your head tilted forward for long periods—which many of us do without realizing it—can make the splenii tight and sore. To ease that tension, tuck your chin in, grasp the back of your head, and gently exert forward pressure.

The trapezius muscle is the large coat-hanger–shaped muscle that links your shoulders to your head. You can find the top of the trapezius by feeling the muscular ridges on your shoulders, just to the right and left of your neck. Anyone who chronically holds his arms in an elevated position—while typing, reading, drawing, or operating machinery, for instance—is a prime candidate for "trapeziitis."

To release the tension, sit in a chair and grip the seat with your left hand, to stabilize your shoulders. With your right hand, bend your head slowly to the right. Repeat on the other side.

Finally, we have the scalene muscles, located just

above the collarbone, deep inside. They are called the "great foolers" because when they start to act up, they can mimic symptoms of a pinched nerve and whiplash, causing pain or numbness in the thumb, the forefinger, the back of the arm, or the shoulder-blade area.

To relax the scalenes, grip the bottom of your chair with your left hand as before. Place your right hand atop your head and pull your head gently to the right. As you do so, guide your head slightly backward. Repeat on the other side.

This last was the stretch the violinist needed. That, and taking a break during practicing her lessons now and then.

Wrist and Forearm Relaxer

I remember once cutting through a ½-inch bolt with a hacksaw. As I slashed away, I suddenly realized that I was gripping the handle much harder than necessary. My forearm ached. All I needed to do was use the proper sawing motion, involving my pectorals, and the job would soon be done. Proper form and a light touch are best.

I was overworking the wrist extensor on top of the forearm. It can cause wrist pain and even mimic tennis elbow. Typists can easily overwork these muscles by keeping their arms frozen over a keyboard much of the day.

Stretch your arm straight out. Bend your wrist down and extend your fingers, pointing to the floor. Twist your hand to the outside, while pressing down and in with your other hand. Repeat with your other hand.

Loosen the Lower You

Finally, here's a stretch with some anthropological interest: the Oriental Squat. It can ease chronic calf pain in runners and stretch the hips and deep tendons of the back. It'll also make it easier to scrounge around under the kitchen sink looking for the cleanser.

With your feet about 12 inches apart, squat down on

217
■

your haunches. Fold your arms and rest them on your knees to maintain balance. Your feet should be slightly turned out, with your heels on the floor.

If you're the average Westerner, you won't care to squat for very long. But in the Far East and elsewhere, it's a position of comfort. African tribesmen have been observed to squat like this for hours, waiting for game.

Taking the Pinch out of Your Buttocks

Imagine that you're washing dishes and standing a good bit away from the sink to avoid splashing yourself. If, in this stance, you were to pick up a heavy frying pan (something I don't recommend), you would feel pressure in the glutei muscles of the buttocks. Besides lifting, the glutei come in for a lot of work during walking and running.

The glutei extend and rotate the thigh and help support the back. When stressed, they can trigger a pain that mimics the irritating jolt of sciatica.

A wonderful stretch for the glutei is the posture Westerners most associate with yoga: the Twist.

The Twist is normally done on the floor, but here is a simpler version you can do in your chair. Place your left leg over the right, and hook your right arm around your left knee to stabilize your legs. Hold on to the chair with your left hand and slowly turn to the left, while exhaling. You should feel a stretch in the left buttock. Repeat on the other side.

Here is another, even simpler version of the Twist. Prop your right foot up on a secure chair or stool, bend your right knee, and slowly move your left shoulder toward your right knee. Breathe out and enjoy the twist. Repeat on the opposite side.

Loosening Your Chest and Arms

Most things we do tend to happen in front of our head. So the arm flexors—the pectorals, biceps, and coracobrachialis muscles—get quite a workout. Athletes sometimes overdevelop these muscles while ignoring the upper back, resulting in round-shoulderedness. That can tilt the head forward and compromise the trapezius. People need to expand and stretch the chest area.

Yoga enthusiasts accomplish it with a pose called (for reasons unclear to me) the Cow Head: They stretch the right hand up and over the right shoulder, work the left hand behind and under the left shoulder, and clasp hands behind their back. Fairly difficult; in fact, I can't even do it. But anyone can do the doorway stretch.

Stand with your hands at shoulder height. Place one hand on each side of a doorway, or the walls in a corner—whichever is more convenient. Your feet should be just far out enough so you can lean into space before you and feel a good stretch in your pectoral muscles. Vary the stretch by raising your hands and placing your forearms on the doorway or walls and again leaning inward.

Above the pecs is the coracobrachialis, consisting of long, thin fibers that help move the arm. If you've ever sat too low while doing "flys" on a Nautilus machine, you've overworked these fellows.

To stretch, reach straight ahead with your right hand and grip the side of the door, with your thumb pointed to the floor. Straighten your elbow. Now, turn your body 180 degrees so your right arm is extended directly behind you. Repeat with your left arm. This also helps to stretch the biceps fully.

Keep a Cold from Migrating 28

Can't shake your head cold? Still sniffling a tissue-box-and-a-half later, long after a cold's usual one-week run? Time to suspect it isn't just a head cold anymore. Or, maybe—just maybe—it wasn't a cold in the first place.

The old adage that a head cold lasts a week if you treat it and seven days if you don't still rings true (give or take a few days), doctors tell us. Ditto for the flu. Antibiotics do nothing to soften the blow of a virus, the cause of both. Cold and flu remedies, however, can help lessen the severity of an attack and, in some cases, may prevent an extended siege. That's because sinuses that are not encouraged to drain or chest congestion that doesn't yield to a good cough can set you up for sinus, ear, or lung infections—and week two of misery.

Sinuses under Siege

An estimated 1 to 5 percent of adult head colds leave sinusitis in their wake. During a cold, the already-narrow sinus passages become inflamed and swollen, impeding the flow of mucus. If the sinuses don't drain, bacteria that are normally escorted out through these passages suddenly find themselves captive; with no way out, they multiply and invade the sinus membrane lining.

The resulting sinus infection is a major pain in the face (over and/or under your eyes). Like a cold, infected sinuses may send you into an "altered state," stealing your sense of smell and deepening your voice. Other telltale signs are stabbing headache, clogged nose, postnasal drip, or fever that outlasts a head cold's usual seven- to ten-day course.

To prevent your cold from running amok in your sinuses, take aspirin or ibuprofen to reduce inflammation and drink lots and lots and *lots* of liquids to "thin" the mucus and ease drainage. (For more tips to unclog a stuffy nose, see "Cold Comfort" on page 222.) If you suspect that your sinuses are under siege, see your doctor immediately. While viral infections can be helped symptomatically, an infection that's bacterial requires prescription antibiotics. Jack M. Gwaltney, Jr., M.D., warns that untreated infection can turn into chronic sinusitis, permanently damaging your sinuses and sometimes requiring surgery to rebuild the drainage system. Although it's very rare, lingering infections inside your head can make their way into your brain, causing meningitis or brain abscess, says Dr. Gwaltney, head of epidemiology and virology at the University of Virginia School of Medicine in Charlottesville.

Now Hear This

Like sinuses, your ears are connected by passageways, called eustachian tubes, to the head-cold zone. Inflamed mucous membranes can swell and close these passages and trap bacteria. It's also possible that overeager nose blowing could turn a cold into an ear infection by blowing the bugs out to your ears, says Dr. Gwaltney.

If you suspect otitis (that's medicalese for ear infection), follow the preceding cold-care advice; that is, take anti-inflammatory drugs and drink plenty of water. In addition, go easy on the nose blowing. Although ear infections can be viral, the vast majority are bacterial in nature.

Mild earaches that come and go during the course of a cold are fairly common and don't necessarily signal an infection. But if the pain in your ear is more than mere discomfort and you're running a low-grade fever—or if the earache gets worse or lasts for more than one day—head for a doctor. Untreated, infection pressure can rupture your eardrum, causing great pain and possibly damaging your hearing.

Chest Cold or Bronchitis?

A good clue that you've got bronchitis and not just a chest cold is that the symptoms appear or continue after the normal ten-day time span. Bronchitis—a secondary infection—means your head cold has headed south into the air tubes deep in your chest—the very last stop before the spongy tissue of your lungs.

Bronchitis is more likely to bloom in your lungs if you smoke, have allergies, or inhale dust and fumes on the job.

If your cold develops into bronchitis, your cough will rock the Richter scale and you'll bring up greenish yellow

221

COLD COMFORT

Some state-of-the-art cold-treatment advice: Tailor your remedies to your symptoms. To help you, here are some suggestions from Thomas A. Gossel, Ph.D., pharmacology department chair at Ohio Northern University.

Stuffy nose. Sip chicken soup or linger in a steamy shower. The fluids you drink or inhale dilute the mucus in your nose and upper throat to help make breathing easier. Use a sleep-inducing decongestant for no more than five days to avoid reinflaming tissues. Avoid oral decongestants if you have high blood pressure.

Runny nose. Use a decongestant spray when your nose won't stop running. Then switch to an oral decongestant. (Follow the decongestant precautions mentioned above.)

By the way, there's no reason to shun milk as "mucus-making" during a head cold. No connection emerged between the amount of milk drunk and mucus produced in 51 cold-burdened people studied at the University of Adelaide, Australia.

phlegm and feel feverish. Sometimes bronchitis clears up on its own. But if it's severe, see a doctor.

Experts suggest using aromatic menthol products like rubs or cough drops, inhaling steam, and drinking plenty of fluids to help combat chest congestion. (Experts caution, however, that oily menthol rubs should be applied only to the outside of the nose, not the inside.)

If you have asthma, you should be aware, too, that a cold can trigger an attack, says Sidney Friedlaender, M.D., clinical professor of medicine at the University of Florida School of Medicine, Gainesville. The trouble is, it may be difficult to distinguish the symptoms. Typically,

Headache, muscle aches, fever. Choose aspirin, acetaminophen, or ibuprofen for adults, but for children and teenagers, avoid aspirin.

Sore throat. Gargle with salt water (1 teaspoon per pint of water) and suck on lozenges. Aim a medicated spray at the back of your throat.

Productive cough. Coughing expels something you need to get out of your chest. So use cough suppressants only if your doctor approves, and avoid them entirely if you have chronic bronchitis or emphysema.

Dry (hacking) cough. Use a suppressant when this kind of cough interferes with your sleep. Expectorants can help you bring up something that's stuck in your chest. Take a full glass of water with each dose of expectorant.

Malaise. Often caused by dehydration during a cold. Dr. Gossel recommends drinking 8 to 12 glasses of water a day.

an asthma attack differs from a cold in the following ways:

■ Wheezing

■ Difficulty breathing air out

■ A cough—either productive or dry—that cough syrups don't quell

■ Breathing problems that hang on more than ten days or keep coming back

See a doctor immediately if you develop these symptoms. Of course, coldlike symptoms are sometimes signs of something else—perhaps another illness that requires different treatment. How do you know? One clue is if it lasts longer than a week and doesn't exhibit any of the complications listed earlier. Often, however, the sooner the problem is diagnosed and treated, the better. That's why it's important to be alert to the subtle differences from day one of your "cold's" onset. You could be facing one of these:

Strep Throat ▶ Think strep when a sore throat hits hard and fast, says infectious disease specialist Alan Bisno, M.D. While strep and colds both bring fever, fatigue, and achiness, strep almost never gives adults a stuffy, runny nose and cough like head colds do. Persistent runny nose is often a sign of strep in infants and small children.

If you suspect strep, see a doctor right away, says Dr. Bisno, professor of medicine at the University of Miami School of Medicine and chief of the medical service at Miami Veterans Affairs Medical Center. A doctor can swab your throat for evidence of streptococcus bacteria (strep throat's cause and namesake) and prescribe a course of appropriate antibiotics. (Incidentally, on rare occasions, the culprit behind a severe sore throat is a noncold virus, such as the one that causes infectious mononucleosis.)

An Allergy ▶ Sneezy nose and itchy throat and eyes score one point for allergy, while colds rate high for blocking up your nose. Allergies drizzle thin and watery mucus, but a cold's mucus thickens and turns yellow or green. Finally, symptoms going strong beyond the ten-day cold limit may mean allergy.

Suspect allergy between spring and fall when trees, grass, and weeds spew allergy-triggering pollen, says Dr. Friedlaender. Look for symptoms to return at the same time each year and plague others around you, especially family members, since allergies can be inherited.

If you think you've discovered an allergy, Dr. Friedlaender says it's safe to try an OTC antihistamine. For daytime, Dr. Friedlaender recommends a product con-

224
■

taining chlorpheniramine because it doesn't have the same drowsiness potential as other antihistamines. Take it 20 to 30 minutes before you go outdoors. If OTCs don't help, check with your doctor about prescription allergy medications.

Pneumonia ▶ Watch for sharp chest pains, vicious cough, waves of chills, and a temperature as high as 105°F. Pneumonia can progress quickly, so get to the doctor fast if you have reason to suspect it. In pneumonia, strep bacteria or a noncold virus manages to slip past your nose, throat, and bronchial tubes and land in your lungs. There, inflammation creates fluid that blankets your lungs' tiny air sacs, blocking the flow of vital oxygen into your body.

Besides prescribing medication, your doctor will tell you to rest in bed and may give you oxygen to inhale if your breathing is too bad. If you are over 50, have diabetes, or heart, kidney, or lung disease, or show any sign of worsening, your doctor will admit you to a hospital for treatment.

Preventing Viral Ping-Pong

It's true that many cold viruses set up an immune reaction in your body that closes the door to reinfection by the same bug. But some viruses may make the rounds of family and friends and then reinfect you.

To ensure a swift recovery from the first round and prevent a second bout, keep your natural defense system strong by heeding the following advice.

Rest ▶ Experts say that even for a common cold, resting in bed for a day or two may head off a head cold's worst.

Eat Nutritiously ▶ Don't starve a cold, but let your appetite be your guide for the first five days. After that, if you're still not hungry, it's time to try forcing small amounts of food.

225

Walk ▶ Moderate exercise may bolster immunity and is safe after the worst of your cold is over, usually after day four. Exercise can worsen a noncold virus, however. Your rule of thumb: Exercise if your symptoms are all above the neck—sneezing, runny nose, and scratchy throat; rest instead if your symptoms are below the neck—fever, muscle aches, appetite loss, and productive, hacking cough.

Restrict Germs ▶ This reduces the chances of a cold making the rounds and then returning to you. Here's how.

■ Set aside your own drinking and eating utensils, even your own telephone if possible.

■ Designate your own bathroom cup and towel.

■ Wash your hands often, preferably with liquid soap since germs may survive on bar soap.

■ Use disposable tissues and throw used ones into the trash.

29   Update on Strep Infections

When Jim Henson died suddenly, the world mourned the tragic loss of the quiet Muppeteer who created Bert, Ernie, Big Bird, Kermit the Frog, and the other lovable Muppets of "Sesame Street." His death also raised an alarming question: Because the pneumonia he succumbed to was caused by group-A streptococcus—the same type of bacteria that causes strep throat in more than ten million people each year—could strep throat possibly be fatal, too?

"What happened to Jim Henson was a rare occurrence, and it's extremely unlikely that the average person who gets strep throat will die from it," says Edward Kaplan, M.D., professor of pediatrics at the University of Minnesota Medical Center in Minneapolis and director of the World Health Organization's Collaborating Center for Reference and Research on Streptococci. But dismissing strep throat as a minor illness can be a serious mistake, he cautions. Some strep throat infections can cause scarlet fever, and if left untreated, the condition can progress to kidney disease or rheumatic fever. In addition, authorities say that in recent years, group-A strep bacteria seem to have become more virulent, and as a result, the infections caused by this type of bacteria have become more common and severe. "No strep infection, including strep throat, should be ignored," says Dr. Kaplan.

Strep Throat Symptoms

Anyone can get strep throat, but the infection most frequently strikes children between the ages of 5 and 15, according to Elsa Suh, M.D., a strep researcher and pediatric cardiologist who specializes in rheumatic heart disease at Rockefeller University in New York City. In both adults and children, strep throat typically causes a sore throat, white pus spots in the throat, sudden fever, and swelling of the lymph glands under the jaw joints. (The nasal congestion and runny nose associated with colds and flu do not usually occur with strep throat.)

"The symptoms may be debilitating or hardly noticeable," Dr. Suh says. "The sore throat, for example, may be mild or severe." Fever can vary between 100° and 104°F, but a child with a high temperature will not feel as sick as an adult with the same fever.

To diagnose strep throat, a physician rubs the lining of the throat with a cotton swab, then does a test for the presence of the strep bacteria. Once an infection is confirmed, an injection of penicillin is administered or a ten-day course of penicillin in pill form is prescribed. (Those allergic to penicillin are usually given erythromycin.)

"Antibiotics relieve the symptoms after a day or two," Dr. Kaplan says, "but it's important to take all the medicine over the entire ten-day period to completely eradicate the infection."

Strep throat can develop any time of the year, but for reasons unknown it typically occurs in the fall, winter, and early spring. The infection is transmitted in respiratory droplets exhaled, coughed, or sneezed by those who harbor the bacteria in their throat.

Dangerous Complications of Strep Throat

Rheumatic fever, which is among the conditions that untreated strep throat can lead to, is a potentially fatal form of heart disease. Anyone can develop it, but school-age children are most susceptible. The disease typically develops a few weeks after strep throat symptoms have cleared up. A red rash and a painful form of arthritis that affects the ankles, knees, hips, shoulders, elbows, and wrists are among rheumatic fever's symptoms. It also may cause serious impairment of the heart's pumping ability, with symptoms including chest pain, fatigue upon minor exertion, swelling of the feet, and rapid pulse and breathing.

Rheumatic fever can be treated with penicillin and anti-inflammatory medications, including aspirin and steroids. However, some victims may suffer permanent damage to the valves that control blood flow through the heart. Sometimes open-heart surgery must be performed, even on children, to replace the damaged valves.

"Once people have had rheumatic fever," Dr. Suh says, "they're likely to get it again if they ever develop another strep infection." To prevent new strep infections and recurrences of rheumatic fever, those who have had the ailment must be given penicillin preventively on a regular basis, possibly for the rest of their life.

"Rheumatic fever is the leading cause of heart disease in children and young adults around the world," says epidemiologist Benjamin Schwartz, M.D., an infectious disease specialist in the Respiratory Diseases Branch of the Centers for Disease Control (CDC) in Atlanta. "It was quite common in this country in the 1800s, but for reasons we can't fully explain, it started tapering off in the United States around 1900, and the decline accelerated after 1960. It became rare here after 1970, and scientists began calling rheumatic fever a 'disease of the past.' But since 1985, clusters of cases have been reported in Missouri, Ohio, and Pennsylvania, and at a military base in California and a children's hospital in Utah. Rheumatic fever may be turning into a real problem again, because of the recent increase in virulence of group-A strep."

Kidney disease, another potential complication of untreated strep throat, develops one to six weeks after strep throat symptoms have disappeared. Symptoms of kidney disease include decreased urination, blood in the urine, which causes darkening of its color, fluid retention (edema), increased blood pressure, and in severe cases, persistent headache and visual disturbances. Poststrep kidney disease is treated with antibiotics and diuretics to decrease fluid retention. The vast majority of children recover completely, but adults who contract poststrep kidney disease may suffer permanent kidney damage.

Strep throat can also cause scarlet fever, which owes its name to the symptoms it causes: red ("strawberry") tongue and a bright red, sandpapery rash on the body, in addition to fever and other strep throat symptoms. Previous strep infections increase susceptibility to scarlet fever, but the condition is successfully treated with antibiotics. Without treatment, however, scarlet fever can lead to such complications as rheumatic fever and kidney disease.

From Colonial times until after the Civil War, scarlet fever was a major childhood killer, Dr. Schwartz says, but the combination of antibiotics and a decline in the virulence of group-A strep bacteria in the past 50 years has reduced it to a minor illness. But now that group-A strep bacteria are becoming more virulent again, "it's possible there will be a rise in cases of scarlet fever, as well as more severe symptoms and a higher incidence of complications from it," says Dennis L. Stevens, M.D., chief of the Infectious Disease Department at the Veterans Affairs Medical Center in Boise, Idaho.

Protect Yourself—Act Fast!

The best way to avoid the dangerous complications of strep throat is to consult your doctor any time you have symptoms that suggest strep throat—especially if you've heard of outbreaks in your community, including those in your child's school or day-care center.

A fast, inexpensive strep test recently approved for doctors is being simplified for home use by microbiologist Vincent Fischetti, Ph.D., an associate professor in the Laboratory of Bacteriology at Rockefeller University. The kit, which could be available within a year or two, would enable people to test themselves or their children at home, making a doctor visit necessary only if the test proved positive. However, the American Academy of Pediatrics has raised strong objections, fearing that tests mistakenly deemed negative could cause people to carry strep infections around for days and unknowingly endanger their health.

To aid in the battle against strep, an experimental vaccine that protects mice from the 30 strains of group-A strep most likely to lead to rheumatic fever has been developed by Dr. Fischetti. "There are so many group-A strep bacteria that, as recently as five years ago, a vaccine seemed impossible," he explains. "But using new laboratory techniques, we've been able to create a vaccine against the most dangerous group-A strains. We hope to test it on humans in about one to two years, and be able to market it in the not-too-distant future."

Deadly New Strains of Strep

The rise in lethal types of group-A strep has experts worried. While there are close to a dozen different groups of strep bacteria, according to CDC strep specialist Dr. Schwartz, group-A strep is causing the most concern. Until recently, he explains, the more than 80 strains in this group primarily caused strep throat, impetigo (a skin condition), and tonsillitis. But group-A strep bacteria as a whole have apparently become more dangerous in recent years, and some data suggest there's been an increase in the incidence and severity of common strep infections. In addition, a few particularly virulent strains have led to a rise in such rare strep diseases as the pneumonia Jim Henson developed. Some of these strains have also caused a new, potentially fatal illness, a toxic-shock–like syndrome. There's concern that other strains of group-A strep may lead to even more new deadly strep-related diseases.

Here are illnesses linked to group-A strep.

Pneumonia ▶ This potentially fatal respiratory illness can occur as a complication of the flu. Young children, the elderly, and those with chronic respiratory ailments are the most likely to be victims. What happened to Jim Henson was so astonishing not only because his pneumonia was caused by group-A strep—a rare occurrence—but also because, other than having a minor cold, he was healthy when the illness struck. And while it typically takes more than a week for untreated pneumonia to prove fatal, Henson died 3½ days after first developing symptoms. "Jim Henson's death was caused by a very toxic, rapidly progressive pneumonia," says David M. Gelmont, M.D., director of medical intensive care at New York Hospital in New York City and the doctor who treated Henson's pneumonia.

"While streptococcal pneumonia is rare, we are seeing more cases of it now, due to the rise in virulent group-A strep strains," says Dr. Kaplan.

Henson's condition could have been treated if it had been caught sooner. But by the time he arrived at the hospital, his organs had begun to shut down due to lack of oxygen from his fluid-filled lungs and the invasion of the strep bacteria into his bloodstream.

Because you can't tell what type of pneumonia you have from the symptoms alone, seek medical treatment immediately for any of the following signs of the illness:

231

■

shortness of breath, difficulty breathing, chest pain, fever, coughing (sometimes accompanied by the spitting up of rust-colored sputum), chills, and headache. A doctor can diagnose bacterial pneumonia with a physical exam and a chest x-ray and treat it with antibiotics.

Toxic-Shock–Like Illness ▶ When toxic-shock syndrome was first identified about ten years ago as a potentially fatal disease in women who'd used super-absorbent tampons, it was caused by staphylococcus ("staph") bacteria, not strep. But more recently, infections caused by a virulent group-A strep strain resulted in about 20 cases and 9 deaths from a toxic-shock–type illness in Colorado. Around that time, Dr. Stevens documented 20 additional cases in otherwise healthy young people in the Rocky Mountain area. "In about half the cases, the strep bacteria entered a break in the skin," says Dr. Stevens. Six of the victims died.

Signs of this new strep-caused toxic-shock–like illness include flulike symptoms, including high fever, debilitating weakness, and aches and pains. If you develop such symptoms, see a doctor promptly. Wash cuts and burns thoroughly and keep them covered. "If the area becomes very red or swollen or increasingly painful, seek medical care immediately," says Dr. Stevens.

Bacterial Septicemia ▶ Group-A strep bacteria can also infect the bloodstream, resulting in bacterial septicemia (blood poisoning). While septicemia usually occurs in the elderly and chronically ill, there is concern that it may become more common as group-A strep bacteria become more virulent. At least 70 cases occurred in Denver alone between January and August 1989. And septicemia caused by the new strains of group-A strep carries an especially high risk of fatality, according to Dr. Stevens.

Symptoms of bacterial septicemia include fever, chills, malaise, and muscle weakness. If a blood test for the strep bacteria is positive, hospitalization and the administration of intravenous antibiotics are required.

Impetigo ▶ If strep bacteria infect an insect bite, cut, or other skin wound, the result can be a skin disease known as impetigo. Symptoms include pain, warmth, redness, swelling, and yellowish pus that forms crusts around the wound. Mild impetigo is treated by washing the affected area with soap and water and applying antibacterial ointment. Severe impetigo requires oral antibiotics. Impetigo is usually not dangerous, but it can progress to toxic-shock–like illness.

Tonsillitis ▶ In many cases, strep throat also infects the tonsils. Symptoms are the same as those of strep throat, but in addition, the tonsils become enlarged and inflamed. If a throat culture indicates strep tonsillitis, penicillin or other antibiotics will be prescribed. If left untreated, the infection may lead to rheumatic fever or kidney disease.

Sinus Infection ▶ Usually a complication of colds and the flu, bacterial sinus infections can be caused by a variety of microorganisms, among them group-A and other types of strep bacteria. This infection causes nasal congestion, runny nose, and pain across the bridge of the nose. Anyone who has these symptoms on a recurring basis should see his or her physician. Bacterial sinusitis is treated with antibiotics. Untreated strep sinusitis can lead to rheumatic fever and kidney disease.

The Science
of
Positive
Living

Heart to Heart 30

By Dean Ornish, M.D.

We know that the traditional risk factors—cholesterol, blood pressure, age, gender, genetics, smoking, diabetes, obesity, sedentary life—explain only about 50 percent of heart disease. At least half of the reasons why people get heart disease are unknown. So why is it that some people get heart disease while others don't? Clearly, all of these risk factors are important, but I don't think that any of them go to the core of why people develop heart disease.

Are there common psychological—and perhaps even spiritual—factors that lead to coronary heart disease?

In the 1950s, Dr. Meyer Friedman and Dr. Ray Rosenman described a syndrome they termed type-A behavior that they believed caused heart disease. The type-A syndrome describes someone who is hostile, self-involved, impatient, and always in a hurry. Type A's make obsessive attempts to achieve poorly defined goals and have a strong need for recognition and advancement. They have a tendency to do two or three things at the same time, such as talking and moving quickly, and so on. At first, studies indicated that type-A behavior was linked with heart disease; later, more conclusive studies failed to substantiate this connection.

Revealing Research

More recent evidence has helped to explain this discrepancy. Research by Dr. Larry Scherwitz at the University of California, San Francisco, Dr. Redford Williams at Duke University, and others indicates that certain elements of type-A behavior are linked with heart disease, whereas other components are not. In particular, the factors most toxic to the heart are self-involvement, hostility, and cynicism.

Dr. Scherwitz, Dr. Lynda Powell, and others found

235
■

that the frequency with which a person refers to himself or herself—that is, how frequently he or she used the words "I," "me," "my," and "mine" in an ordinary conversation—actually predicted the recurrence of a heart attack. The more frequently a person used these words, the greater the likelihood he or she would die from a heart attack.

In another study, Dr. Scherwitz analyzed tape-recorded interviews from a nine-year research study involving almost 13,000 men. This study, called the Multiple Risk Factor Intervention Trial (MRFIT), was designed to determine if moderate lifestyle changes could help prevent heart disease. Dr. Scherwitz found that people who used frequent self-references later developed heart disease more often than people who didn't. Most striking was the even greater degree of self-involvement in those who ultimately died from heart attacks.

Well, why should that be true? Certainly, saying the words, "I," "me," "my," and "mine" isn't harmful per se. Instead, our speech reflects how we view the world we live in. When we feel isolated from others, we focus more on ourselves—"I need this. I want that."

These research studies have taken us a major step in the right direction, but they raise even more basic questions. I wonder: Why are we self-involved? Why are we cynical? Why are we hostile? Is there a more fundamental cause for these emotions that can lead to coronary heart disease and other illnesses?

I believe that there is. Living with patients for a month at a time in our earlier studies and meeting with them frequently and intensively during the past four years of our third study has provided me with some special opportunities. At first I viewed our support groups simply as a way to motivate patients to stay on the other aspects of the program that I considered most important: the diet, exercise, stress-management training, stopping smoking, and so on.

Over time, I began to realize that the group support itself was one of the most powerful interventions, as it addressed what I am beginning to believe is a more fundamental cause of why we feel stressed and, in turn, why we get illnesses like heart disease: the perception of isolation.

In short, anything that promotes a sense of isolation leads to chronic stress and often to illnesses like heart disease. Conversely, anything that leads to real intimacy and feelings of connection can be healing in the real sense of the word: to bring together, to make whole. The ability to be intimate has long been seen as a key to emotional health; I believe it is essential to the health of our heart as well.

The Risk of the Lonely Heart

I wrote *Stress, Diet, and Your Heart* in 1982. When I conducted the two earlier studies that formed the basis of that book, I was only beginning to explore these ideas. There was not much scientific literature at that time to support my clinical observations. Since then, though, increasing scientific evidence is demonstrating that isolation and suppression of feelings often leads to illness, whereas intimacy and social support can be healing. Let's examine a few of these studies.

■ In the Alameda County Study (6,928 men and women living near San Francisco) and in the North Karelia Study (13,301 men and women living in eastern Finland) participants were studied for five to nine years. Those who were socially isolated had a twofold to threefold increased risk of death from both heart disease and from all other causes when compared with those who felt most connected to others. These results were independent of other cardiac risk factors, such as cholesterol level, blood pressure, genetics, and so on. Similar results were found in 2,059 subjects from Evans County, Georgia, where the greatest mortality was found in older people with few social ties.

Even being a member of a club, church, or synagogue significantly decreased the risk of premature death and significantly protected people from heart dis-

237
■

ease even when they had high blood pressure. In a subsequent nine-year period, those whose social connections decreased experienced a greater risk of death from heart disease.

■ Studies by other investigators have shown that people who live alone have more heart disease than those who live with someone or even something—a plant or a pet, even a goldfish. So being the petter or the pettee has many health benefits, probably because it decreases isolation.

■ At Yale University School of Medicine, scientists studied 119 men and 40 women who were undergoing coronary angiography. They found that the more people felt loved and supported, the less coronary atherosclerosis they had at angiography, independent of other risk factors such as age, sex, income, hypertension, serum cholesterol, smoking, diabetes, genetics, and hostility.

■ In one study reported by Dr. William Ruberman in the *New England Journal of Medicine,* interviews with 2,320 male survivors of heart attacks revealed that patients who were classified as being socially isolated and having a high degree of life stress had more than four times the risk of death from heart disease and from all other causes when compared with men who had low levels of both stress and isolation.

■ At the Medical College of Wisconsin, Dr. James Goodwin and his colleagues found that unmarried persons with cancer had decreased overall survival, even after adjustment for disease severity and type of treatment. In another study, he found that among 256 healthy elderly adults, individuals with good social support systems tended to have lower blood cholesterol levels and higher indices of immune function. These findings were independent of age, smoking, alcohol intake, and degree of emotional stress.

■ A report published in the journal *Science* reviewed the mounting evidence that social isolation heightens people's susceptibility to illness. According to Dr. James House, one of the authors of the report, "It's the 10 to 20 percent of people who say they have nobody with whom they can share their private feelings, or who have close contact with others less than once a week, who are at most risk."

The report said that "social isolation is as significant to mortality rates as smoking, high blood pressure, high cholesterol, obesity, and lack of physical exercise. In fact, when age is adjusted for, social isolation is as great or greater a mortality risk than smoking. After controlling for the effects of physical health, socioeconomic status, smoking, alcohol, exercise, obesity, race, life satisfaction, and health care, the studies found that those with few or weak social ties were twice as likely to die as those with strong ties." The authors concluded by stating, "Thus, just as we discover the importance of social relationships for health, and see an increasing need for them, their prevalence and availability seem to be declining."

The self-involvement, hostility, and cynicism that predispose us to heart disease are really effects of a more fundamental cause: the perception of isolation. When someone feels isolated and alone, then his focus is on himself: "I feel alone. I am lacking. If only I had _____, then I'd be happy." The perception of isolation leads to self-involvement. Likewise, the chronic frustration and recurrent disappointments and disillusionments of not getting what we think will make us happy—or getting it and finding that the happiness doesn't last—can lead to chronic hostility and cynicism.

When we perceive ourselves only as isolated and alone—apart from the world instead of a part of it—then we are likely to feel chronically stressed. Chronic stress, in turn, can lead to heart disease both in its direct effects on the heart and because of the self-destructive behavior patterns that result. Anything that helps transcend and transform this perceived isolation can be healing.

Healing Communication

How we approach other people each day can determine whether we experience isolation, chronic stress, suffering, and illness, or intimacy, relaxation, joy, and health. Of course, touching, hugging, and massage are ways of increasing intimacy. Here's another powerful technique that can help us to feel more connected to others and to transcend our sense of separateness instead of feeling alone and isolated.

We can learn how to talk to each other in ways that allow the other person to hear us better. When we feel heard, then we feel more connected. And feeling connected and heard is an important part of the healing process because it reduces the feelings of isolation that lead to stress and illness.

Communication and ventilation are not the same. Ventilation is just getting your feelings out; you really don't care whether the person hears you or not. Communication is expressing how you feel to someone so that he or she can hear and understand you better. It's a skill that can be learned.

Many people believe that merely ventilating anger is good for you—a catharsis of negative emotions. But is it? In her book *Anger: The Misunderstood Emotion,* Carol Tavris outlines research that questions this assumption. She writes, "The psychological rationales for ventilating anger do not stand up under experimental scrutiny. The weight of evidence indicates precisely the opposite: Expressing anger makes you angrier, solidifies an angry attitude, and establishes a hostile habit."

Oftentimes it seems that when we're in a relationship with someone—either a work relationship or a personal one—we have to choose between either holding our feelings in and making ourselves increasingly upset or exploding and making others around us angry.

But we have another option: communicating our feelings in ways that are more likely to be heard without causing the other person to feel attacked.

The basic principle of good communication is that our feelings help to connect us, whereas thoughts—especially judgments—tend to isolate us. Our emotions are more likely to be heard by someone than our thoughts. It doesn't always happen that way, but expressing our feelings increases the likelihood that it will.

Communicating ideas brings our minds together, whereas communicating emotions unites our hearts—not quite the same experience. The clear expression of genuine feelings, even negative ones, is a gift to both ourselves and to others, for it helps to bring us together. Thoughts connect our heads, feelings join our hearts. Why?

■ Thoughts are much more likely to be heard as criticisms than are feelings. If one person says, "I think you're wrong," or "I think you're a jerk," then the other person is likely to feel verbally attacked or criticized. At that point, the walls (emotional defenses) go up, the discussion spirals downward, and no one really wins. Both people may start arguing about feeling attacked rather than whatever was originally bothering them.

■ As soon as we feel criticized by someone, it's very hard to hear anything else he or she has to say. If I communicate a feeling instead—"I feel hurt by what you did"—then you're less likely to perceive it as an attack. It's easier for you to hear what I'm saying. Being heard and understood is what we really want.

■ Expressing feelings seems to make us a little vulnerable, although it really makes us safer. Part of what makes being in a close relationship with someone feel so scary is that we know each other's soft spots very well. No one else knows how to hurt us quite as effectively. When we're feeling attacked or judged by a friend, family member, or loved one, the human tendency is to want to attack back and go right for the soft underbelly. But when we communicate our feelings, then we're exposing part of ourselves to the other person. And when you make yourself a little more vulnerable, your heart a little more open, then it makes it easier for the other person to respond in kind. It helps both people feel safer and thus more free.

Talking Your Way to Closeness 241

■

The basic principles of these communication skills are fairly simple, but it takes a lot of practice before they become a habit. At first, the distinction between thoughts and feelings may seem like splitting hairs, but it makes an important difference in how well we communicate. These techniques can be used for expressing—and receiving—positive feelings as well as negative ones. Here's how it's done.

Step 1: Identify What You Are Feeling ▶ This isn't as easy as it sounds. Many people have a hard time telling the difference between a thought and a feeling. What are some common feelings?

- I'm angry.
- I'm afraid.
- I'm worried.
- I'm thrilled.
- I'm confused.
- I'm happy.
- I'm depressed.
- I'm envious.
- I'm resentful.
- I love you.
- I want _____.

What are some common thoughts or judgments?

- I'm right.
- You're wrong.
- You're not listening.
- You did it again.
- You're always late.
- You're a jerk (always a subject for intense debate).
- You forgot.
- You should wear different clothes.

Sometimes thoughts masquerade as feelings:

- I feel that I'm right.
- I feel as if you're wrong.

- I feel you should do it better.
- I feel you ought to be more careful.

Using the words "that," "like," or "as if" after "I feel" is a clue that what follows is probably a thought (a judgment), not a feeling. Words like "you should," "you ought to," "you never," and "you always" are thoughts and are almost always heard as judgments or criticisms.

Step 2: Express What You Are Feeling ▶ Say exactly how you feel, but express it as a feeling rather than as a thought or judgment. You don't have to tone it down, make it nice, or pretend. It is as important to express negative feelings as positive ones, but express them as feelings and information rather than as judgments and criticisms.

Communicating your feelings is not a panacea, but it does help to break the vicious circle of attack, counterattack, and withdrawal. It's not going to solve all your problems, but at least it won't add more problems to the ones you already have. You can begin to focus on the real issues and deal with those instead of arguing about the arguing and fighting about the fighting. As a result, each person is more likely to get what he or she wants.

Step 3: Listen Actively with Empathy and Compassion ▶ Knowing how to listen is as important a communication skill as knowing how to express feelings. Try to hear the feeling in what the other person is saying, even if he or she is not expressing it clearly or is expressing it as a judgment.

Remember that the other person wants to feel heard, just as you do. You're not always going to get the other person to agree with you, but at least you'll understand each other better. Opening, listening, and giving one's attention help to bring us together. Compassion and empathy are healing.

Empathy is not the same as sympathy. Empathy means listening with compassion—trying to experience and understand what the other person is feeling. Sym-

243

pathy means feeling sorry for someone, a usually well-intentioned gesture that often creates more distance between two people. The unspoken message can be, "You're the one with the problem, not me."

A variant of sympathy is giving unsolicited advice. When we hear someone describing a problem, our tendency is to try to "fix" it by jumping in with our own advice, comments, criticisms, or experiences. Often the other person just wants to feel listened to and understood, which leads to greater intimacy even when the problem is not easily solvable.

The unspoken message behind unsolicited advice can be, "I know the answer; how come you don't?" This creates more distance and less intimacy. Listening is very often a more supportive response than giving someone advice.

Step 4: Acknowledge What the Other Person Is Saying ▶ Expressing that you understand what the other person is saying is not the same as agreeing with it. For example, you might say, "I understand that you're feeling angry because I got home late. And I'm frustrated because I wanted to be home with you, but I had to stay late to finish that report."

It's easier to acknowledge feelings than thoughts or judgments. If someone says to me, "I feel angry," it's a lot easier to acknowledge that feeling than if he says, "You're always late for dinner." And it's easier to apologize when someone expresses hurt or angry feelings than if that person attacks or judges us.

To make this less abstract, here's a real-life example from a group session with Joe and Anita Cecena, tape-recorded at one of our research group meetings

JOE: You went to the store today and spent too much money, Anita. How come?

DEAN: Is what you expressed a thought or a feeling?

JOE: A thought.

DEAN: Anita, how do you feel when he says that?

ANITA: Criticized. Attacked.

DEAN: What would be your natural inclination to do next?

ANITA: To argue and defend myself. Or to attack back. Usually I just ignore him, just tune him out. Sometimes I pretend I don't hear him. Or I'll say, "Yes, dear," and then do it anyway.

DEAN: Joe, when you feel ignored, how do you respond?

JOE: I feel like I'm losing control. Powerless. Sometimes I feel abandoned. And then I get angry, because I don't like feeling that way.

DEAN: Joe, how else could you express how you feel about Anita's shopping?

JOE: Anita, what did you buy that cost so much?

DEAN: Would you say that's a thought or a feeling?

JOE: A thought, I guess.

DEAN: Anita, do you still feel criticized?

ANITA: Yes—it's a little less harsh than before, but it still leaves me feeling pretty much the same way.

DEAN: Okay, Joe, what is the feeling underlying those thoughts?

JOE: That she's a compulsive spender.

DEAN: Now, is that a thought or a feeling?

JOE: Hmmm . . . a thought.

DEAN: And a judgment.

JOE: What if I say, "I feel like she's a compulsive spender."

DEAN: That's a thought masquerading as a feeling, and I suspect Anita also feels criticized when you say that.

ANITA: Right.

DEAN: When she came back from shopping and told you what she spent, what did you feel? What's the feeling that underlies what you are trying to communicate?

JOE: Anger and frustration. And I'm a little worried that we might not have enough money to pay the rest of our bills.

DEAN: Anita, when you felt criticized by Joe, how did you feel?

ANITA: Angry and frustrated.

245

DEAN: So the irony is that both people end up feeling the same way—in this example, angry, frustrated, misunderstood, with a loss of control—and yet each thinks the other person doesn't understand what he or she is feeling. Neither person feels listened to or understood. This frequently happens in arguments between two people, yet it's the opposite of what they both want. Joe, try expressing your feelings instead of your thoughts to Anita.

JOE: When you bought those gifts, I felt angry and frustrated, and a little worried.

DEAN: Anita, do you feel attacked now?

ANITA: When he says it that way, no, I don't.

DEAN: Do you want to attack back, withdraw, or argue with him?

ANITA: Not now. And I knew when I spent so much money that he'd feel this way. But I feel that Joe tends to be very domineering and controlling.

DEAN: Joe, when Anita says, "I feel that you tend to be very domineering and controlling," how do you feel?

JOE: I feel attacked and misunderstood. And judged.

DEAN: Just like Anita does. Anita, anytime someone says, "I feel that you . . . ," it's probably a thought, not a feeling.

When we're feeling controlled, then attacking the other person is one way to try to rebalance the power in the relationship. And going on the attack does often make the other person feel less in control and more in pain. That may be what we want at the moment, but it's not going to give us what we really want, which is to feel more free and intimate with our partner. So try expressing what you said as a feeling instead of a judgment.

ANITA: Joe, I've been feeling dominated and controlled by you, and as a result I spent the money as a way of trying to feel freer and more independent.

DEAN: This allows both of you to focus on the underlying issues and to address them more directly. Anita, when you said earlier, "You're dominating and controlling me," then you're judging Joe. It puts all of the responsibility and blame on him. Instead, when you now said, "I feel dominated and controlled," it reflects how you're feeling, which takes into account that you may have misperceived him. For example, you may be sensitive to feeling dominated because of bad experiences in prior relationships. Or Joe may, in fact, be dominating you. But expressing the feeling frees both of you to explore a wider range of possibilities.

JOE: Anita, I want you to tell me when you're feeling controlled or manipulated by me, and I'll try to stop doing it.

Saying "I want" is a clear and direct feeling—no one can argue if it's true or not. And it makes you a little more open and vulnerable, since the other person knows he or she can disappoint you by not giving you what you want. But saying "I want" is something most of us are taught not to express. It sounds too demanding. So we often tiptoe around the issue without saying it directly.

In fact, because it is so clear and straightforward, saying "I want" is less likely to make someone else feel manipulated than if you try to get what you want in a more indirect way. And when we feel manipulated or controlled, we don't feel totally free.

Note: You can learn these communication skills on your own, but often you get best results when you acquire these skills with the help of a therapist.

The Healing Power of Visualization   31

After examining you for a drippy head cold, your doctor smiles and says, "Take three images and call me in the morning." What? Has she lost her marbles?

Nope. Not at all. "Mental videos" may very well be one prescription you'll be receiving in the not-too-distant future. Known as "creative imagery" (or visualization), conjuring vivid pictures in the mind is gaining favor as an adjunct therapy for everything from headaches and weight loss to chronic pain, heart disease, and cancer.

Some proponents say that mental images can directly influence bodily processes—like shrinking a cancerous tumor or flushing away a flu virus. Science has yet to substantiate that. It's clear, though, that visualization can influence our health and well-being indirectly—and sometimes powerfully.

There's already evidence that what might be called "behavioral visualization"—seeing in our mind's eye how we want to act—can help us transform behavior. There's also research suggesting that imagery may help us fight disease—or make it easier to endure—by reducing stress and promoting relaxation. And scientists know that imagery does seem to influence the immune system for the better. Whether this influence is powerful enough to change the course of illness is unknown, but it's prompted some experts to combine visualization with traditional therapy.

The best way to understand imagery is to experience it for yourself. Like tasting a banana, one bite of the real thing means more than anything anyone could tell you.

Some of the applications—like imaging for the possible relief of serious diseases like chronic pain or cancer—require professional guidance. And they should always be used as an addition to the standard medical treatment, not as a substitute for it. But other applications are easy to do yourself. You can do them right at home, right away. And if you practice faithfully (by which we mean twice a day), you're likely to reap results within just a few weeks. Here are some of the ways that imagery can help.

Washing Stress Away

Imagery's most universal use is for inducing relaxation, which has health-promoting benefits in itself. "Relaxation is an antidote to stress," says Janice Benjamin, a registered nurse who teaches imagery to patients at the National Institutes of Health's pain research clinic. "You can't be stressed and relaxed at the same time."

Stress causes the fight-or-flight response, the body's physical preparation to cope with what threatens our well-being. Our heart beats faster; hormones flood our system; our breath becomes quick and shallow; we break out in a sweat. In moderation, it's a lifesaving response that helps us move and think fast. But in excess, it overstresses us and can contribute to illness.

Techniques to combat stress are rapidly becoming essential components of treatment in hospitals and clinics across the country. Tension—both muscular and mental—can complicate the treatment of any disease. Relaxation exercises like imagery, deep breathing, progressive muscle relaxation, and meditation help reduce tension and anxiety. In one study, patients who used relaxation techniques to destress prior to surgery had speedier recoveries and less postoperative pain, reduced their medication, and just felt better all around when compared with a group who did nothing.

The link between a person's inability to cope with stress and increased susceptibility to certain diseases has been clearly established in recent years. Heart disease, ulcers, chronic fatigue syndrome, low back ache, breast pain, bruxism, and even bad breath—all are known to be stress related.

Seymour Diamond, M.D., uses imagery exercises extensively with migraine patients at the Diamond Headache Clinic in Chicago. "Most headaches are tension related," he says. "Relaxation, especially before the headache has a chance to get bad, often relieves the muscular tension that contributes to more severe and increased numbers of headaches."

The best type of imagery to induce relaxation is guided imagery, in which a voice (live or recorded) takes you through a scripted sequence of calming images. Nature trips are the most popular. The following is an abbreviated example of a favorite among Dr. Diamond's migraine patients.

"Lie down, close your eyes, and focus on your breath. After a few minutes, begin to imagine being at the beach in exquisite detail. Hear the waves breaking; see the clouds floating by; smell the salty air; feel the breeze brushing your arm.

"As you lie there, become aware of any tension that remains in your body. Picture a tiny, soothing wave the size of your hand rolling up toward the sand and approaching you slowly. Feel the warmth of the water as it enters your body and flows directly to the area of tension. The tiny wave seems to gather up the tension and then slowly recedes, taking the tension out of your body. It flows down the sand and into the ocean, leaving you relaxed."

"Creative imagination leads to the relaxation response when you focus your awareness on soothing sensations and a passive attitude. Then your mind naturally grows quiet," says Margaret Ennis, an instructor in the Behavioral Medicine Clinic at the New England Deaconess Hospital in Boston.

Be sure to take the time to draw on as many senses as possible. "It's fine if the actual mental picture is vague. What's important is to quiet down the mind through focusing on any combination of sensory details—sound, touch, even taste," explains Ennis. "Appreciate and accept what you're experiencing—don't worry about how big the next wave will be." The whole creative imagination sequence could take a few minutes or half an hour.

Retraining your mind to think in positive thoughts and images on a moment-to-moment basis also helps reduce the negative physiological effects of the stress response. "It's the nature of the mind to think and imagine constantly," adds Ennis. "The question is, what are the contents of your thoughts? If negative images are always playing in your mind, you suffer the consequences in your body." The fight-or-flight response is triggered by perception, not reality. "If you see a rope and think it's a snake, your breath will quicken, your heart will race, and you'll break out in a sweat," says Ennis. "But if you see a snake and think it's a rope, your body will be calm."

What that means is that if in your daily life you constantly perceive "snakes," your body will respond accordingly, gearing up physically for fight or flight. Using imagery, you can learn to replace negative images with positive ones and give your body a break from excess stress.

One rule of thumb, though: If an image makes you anxious, don't hesitate to find an alternative that eliminates the source of displeasure.

See It, Then Do It

Imaging for success has been popular for years with Olympic athletes and high-powered business executives, people committed to securing every possible advantage for success. And studies prove that it works: What people are able to see, they're more likely to be able to do.

In one study, college students who were preparing for public speaking significantly reduced their apprehension by using visualization. They were asked to envision the best possible scenario: putting on just the right clothes; feeling clear, confident, and thoroughly prepared; giving a smooth, brilliant speech that was well received. Other stress-reduction techniques, such as muscle relaxation and desensitization, did not work as well.

If imagining a positive outcome promotes success on the playing field or at the podium, is it possible that thinking healthy thoughts might lead to better health? It's only a theory at this point, but some physicians believe it's a distinct possibility.

One firm believer is Errol Korn, M.D., a member of the clinical faculty at the University of California in San Diego. In his opinion, "end-result" imagery can work in any circumstance for anyone who wants to achieve a particular result. Although he now works primarily with businesspeople for enhancing career potential, Dr. Korn has written scripts for numerous guided-imagery cassette tapes ranging from getting a good night's sleep to overcoming overeating to lowering blood pressure.

"All that's needed is to image the desired outcome

exactly how you want it," he says. "And that will be the same for any situation or disease, because everyone wants to become a well, healthy, and functioning human being."

Tapping Your Inner Wisdom

Clinicians at the Behavioral Medicine Clinic integrate imagery into treatment, using it both to elicit the relaxation response and for the reduction of chronic pain.

The mechanisms for registering pain in the body are very complex. One natural human response to pain is to tense around it to protect the area. And when you tighten one place, you tighten others. You end up suffering a lot of secondary pain and tension in addition to the initial pain. This begins a vicious circle of pain and tension. To

FOR PEOPLE WHO SUFFER MIGRAINES: THINK WARM

At the Diamond Headache Clinic in Chicago, migraine patients use imagery to abort headaches. They are trained to close their eyes and vividly picture their hands over a hot fire or radiator. "Raising hand temperature with the mind is very effective," says Seymour Diamond, M.D., director of the clinic. "Why or how, no one knows for sure."

One theory is that it redirects blood flow, diverting blood away from the head to the extremities. Another is that it causes a "neural reflex" in nerves that control the blood vessels in the head. What's curious is that only heat generated by the mind does the trick. When patients' hands are heated by placing them in hot water, headaches aren't affected.

break the cycle, patients can identify the physical and emotional tensions that perpetuate it.

Imaging pictures or symbols of what their pain looks like often offers patients the clues needed to help break the cycle. Under the guidance of the skilled professional, creative imaging exercises combine with talking with the patient to help clarify the nature of the pain, by showing where and how tension is being held in the body. This, in turn, often helps them reduce the pain by giving them a better awareness of how it works. Without awareness you don't have the control that allows change.

For instance, finding a clear image of her migraine pain had a dramatic effect on the life of a woman who'd suffered frequent hospitalization from headaches for over 25 years. "I'd always had the sense that my pain was like a ball in my head," she says. "And when the ball tilted, I knew a doozy was coming. I had no idea, however, that I could control the ball." After this realization, she was able to dramatically reduce the number and severity of her headaches. As soon as she'd feel the ball beginning to tilt, she'd lie down, close her eyes and, through her imagination, take the ball out of her head.

Although it's impossible to know how imagery may have physiologically worked in this case, Ennis speculates that the ball symbolized the muscle tension in the neck and head. By making the visual association, the woman was able to release the tension by getting rid of the ball. Developing that kind of bodily control, however, is no easy task. "There's no language to communicate the how-to to people," says Ennis. "It can only be gained experientially—that is, by trying it over and over again until it works."

Boosting Immunity

The notion that people can use images to mentally "see" their immune system fighting cancer cells has been popular since the 1970s. Reports of success stories and spontaneous remissions abound, but anecdotes alone aren't proof. "It's a controversial area," says Nicholas Hall, Ph.D., director of the Division of Psychoimmunology at the University of South Florida Psychiatry Center. "But the view that the immune system may play a role in combating at least certain kinds of cancer is generally accepted."

Studies suggest that when we're under excess stress, the body releases stress hormones. Chronic high levels of these chemicals can diminish the activity of antibodies and natural killer cells that protect us against foreign invaders and tumors. That depression might lead to increased risks of cancer and other immune-mediated conditions.

Dr. Hall has been involved in several studies that measured the immune functions of cancer patients who practiced relaxation and imagery regularly. In all of the studies to date, significant increases in certain immunologic measurements were seen from before imaging to during imaging.

"Imagery does appear to increase the ability of the immune cells to function," states Dr. Hall. "The question is, 'Is that the way things would have been had the patients not done the imagery?' " No one knows. Although the data show a definite correlation between imaging and improved immunity, cause and effect is hard to establish. Immune factors are constantly fluctuating anyway.

Studies testing mind/body interactions are hard to design because of the many uncontrollable and confounding variables: diet, the placebo effect, exercise, social support, other treatments. All form a complex web of influence. "We haven't yet been clever enough to design the study that would isolate which particulars are working to what degree," says Dr. Hall.

The evidence is too preliminary to make a solid claim about imagery's ability to zap cancer cells. But Dr. Hall believes that doing something that might increase the ability of the immune cells to function, even if it's not directly fighting cancer, could help in resisting other infections.

Stress is unavoidable. Always has been and always will be. But unavoidable doesn't mean unmanageable. The latest stress research shows that how you react to a stressful event is what determines its impact on your health. If you let stress bother you, it *will* bother you, and in ways that can be physical as well as mental. Virtually every organ in the body can be negatively influenced by poorly handled stress.

But handle stress intelligently and you turn the enemy into an ally. Stress can motivate, invigorate, instigate, and educate. It can be a kick in the pants rather than a slap in the face.

The following host of stress busters offers you the chance to discover some personally effective techniques. Some of these antistress strategies get at the causes of stress (which, of course, is the preferred way of beating it). Others give temporary relief by treating its symptoms. Both approaches have their place, and combining them into one double-barreled stratagem may be what it takes to slay the beast.

Not all these techniques are appropriate for everyone. And not all are backed by rock-solid scientific data—a lot of them are just good bets based on common sense. So you'll have to catalog shop, select what you think might work for you, and see what destresses best.

Instant Soothers

For quick, temporary stress relief that takes the edge off the moment, there's a lot you can do. "But stress reduction is a very personal thing, meaning that what works for one person may not work for another," says Paul Rosch, M.D., of the American Institute of Stress. So here are some stress releasers that come with no guarantees but are options that are worth a try when you need to find a little relief in a hurry.

Decompression Breaks ▶ You come home after a bad day feeling as friendly as a wolverine. Do you try to mix with the family "as is"? You might try decompressing first. Go for a walk or take a shower. Do anything to let your mood run out of steam. By leaping right in with the family—dealing too soon with yet another set of concerns and personalities—you could be intensifying your stress. Try decompression breaks at work, too, or any time you feel yourself running too hot. A few minutes to cool down may be all you need.

Humor ▶ Make light of a heavy situation and it immediately loses some of its weight. Comedians have been doing this for us for centuries, says Steven Allen, Jr., M.D. (yes, the son of comic genius Steve Allen), but we need to get better at doing it for ourselves. "We need to revere humor in these high-stress times of ours, not just tolerate it." Try to laugh it up more at work, Dr. Allen says, and look for humorous elements on the home front. Go so far as to imagine how your domestic snags might be handled by the producers of a TV comedy show. There's a little (or a lot) of humor in everything if we can just relax enough to see it.

But sometimes it's tough to force a laugh in tense situations. What do you do? One technique that can help do the trick involves blowing a situation out of proportion—to the point that it becomes laughable. If you're stuck in a traffic jam, for example, construct the worst scenario imaginable. "These cars will never move. I'll be stuck here for the rest of my life. By the time I get out, my children will have grown up, married, and had children of their own. They won't even remember who I am." When your scenario reaches the point of absurdity, you begin to smile at yourself. It puts the situation in perspective, which calms you down.

Pets ▶ We talk to them, we pet them, we cuddle them, we confide in them. Pets, as a result, can be great stress reducers. Some people feel their pet is like a psychiatrist they don't have to pay.

Yes, pet therapy is proving capable of producing many of the same relaxation benefits as other, more conventional forms of treatment. Research has shown that heart attack victims who have pets live longer, that pets can help ease household tensions, and that even just watching a tank full of tropical fish may lower blood pressure, at least temporarily.

Why are pets so soothing?

"Animals bring out our nurturing instinct," says Linda Hines, executive director of the Delta Society, an organization dedicated to studying human/animal interactions. "They also make us feel safe and unconditionally accepted. We can just be ourselves around our pets."

Pets also can help bring out our lighter, more playful side. "Studies show that even people who are normally reserved will loosen up around animals," Hines says. To keep animals from being a source of stress, however, it's important to choose a pet that's not going to take more of your time—or your house—than you have to give.

"It doesn't do any good to get a pet and then feel guilty that you're not giving it enough attention," Hines says.

It's also a good idea to be sure that your pet is housebroken and well trained. "Accidents in the house and annoyed friends and neighbors can be stress makers, not breakers."

Attitude Tune-Ups

Stress for many of us is caused not so much by our environment as by our attitudes. Perhaps you expect too much of yourself or others. Or maybe you suffer from low self-esteem and remain too passive. Either way, stress can result as we fail to get from life what we feel we deserve. The solution?

257

We need to change the attitudes that generate stress in the first place. The following disciplines and techniques are dedicated to doing that.

Assertiveness Training ▶ The secretary who feels like a slave. The sales associate who feels frustrated mired at the bottom of the corporate ladder. Rodney Dangerfield is not alone! What he and these people lack is respect—both from themselves and from others. What they need to turn that around is to be assertive—that is, to be able to communicate needs and feelings.

Here are a few simple principles. Be straightforward: Say no politely and firmly; don't make excuses. Admit your feelings. Say, "I'm angry" rather than, "You make me mad." Express your preferences and priorities: Say, "I don't have a particular movie to suggest, although I do want to avoid ones with violence" instead of, "I don't care—whatever everyone else wants is okay with me." Most experts agree that assertiveness training isn't for everyone, but if you're fearful of rejection and afraid of emotional confrontations, you could be a candidate.

For more information, or to get in touch with a counselor specializing in assertiveness therapy, contact your local mental health organization or the psychology department at a nearby college or university. Or check with your family doctor.

Delegating ▶ Why are some top executives under less stress than many homemakers? Because they've learned to delegate. They've learned the fine art of sharing the load. "Stress for many of us is a self-inflicted burden in this regard," says psychologist Steven Fahrion, Ph.D., of the Menninger Clinic in Topeka, Kansas. Whether because of too much ego, or not enough, we fail to get others to pitch in where they can and should.

This isn't to say we should become dictators, but it does suggest we consider how our time might best be spent. The idea, the experts say, is to delegate what we can so that we're able to spend more time on the things that we can't. We shouldn't feel guilty about passing out responsibilities, because by delegating—to our children, especially—we help others learn self-sufficiency.

Cognitive Therapy ▶ Thoughts cause feelings, and the wrong kind of thoughts can cause stressful feelings. "We cause ourselves a lot of unnecessary anxiety by seeing the glass as half empty rather than as half full," says cognitive therapist and marriage counselor Fran Gaal.

Call it twisted thinking; there are lots of examples. Do you automatically interpret silence on the part of your spouse to mean anger when it could just as easily mean fatigue? Do you blame yourself when a sudden downpour drenches your wash on the line? Do you dwell on the few times your boss criticized your performance and ignore the innumerable times she's praised you?

We all fall into the negative thinking rut from time to time. We may overgeneralize, jump to conclusions, badger ourselves with "should haves," and lose sight of the fact that "good" and "bad" in life is rarely black and white.

"Think in shades of gray," says psychiatrist and cognitive therapist David D. Burns, M.D., "not black or white only." All-or-nothing thinking can lead to anxiety, depression, guilt, feelings of inferiority, perfectionism, and anger.

For more information, especially if you're interested in exploring cognitive therapy more fully, check with your family doctor or local health bureau for someone trained in the discipline. Or consult *The Feeling Good Handbook: Using the New Mood Therapy in Everyday Life* by Dr. Burns.

Support Groups ▶ Misery may like company, but the desire for comfort likes it even more. "Support groups give their members an opportunity to do something about their problems and to be more than passive victims," says John Renner, M.D., president of the Consumer Health Information Research Institute. "They reduce the sense of isolation that people often feel when afflicted with a serious health dilemma."

So whether it's a drug or alcohol problem or an eating disorder, a gambling addiction or a recent divorce, there's a group out there willing to listen and to help alleviate some of the stress.

For more information, or for help in locating such a group, your best bet is to contact a support-group clearinghouse. Two such national organizations are the Self-Help Center, 1600 Dodge Avenue, Evanston, IL 60201, and the National Self-Help Clearinghouse, 25 West 43rd Street, Room 620, New York, NY 10036.

Procrastination Relief ▶ "But I do my best work under pressure."

Baloney, says psychologist Neil Fiore, Ph.D. By putting things off, you wind up having to wrestle with self-disapproval, besides the task at hand. It's a double whammy that can inhibit optimal performance in addition to being unhealthfully stressful. He offers these tips for procrastinators.

Enjoy your playtime guilt-free. Fill your weekly schedule with time for leisure and friends—then watch your resentment toward work melt away. Avoid being overwhelmed by trying to finish. Instead, focus on the key phrase "When can I start?" This puts your mind on small, achievable steps with specific starting times.

Or you can always try what Michael LeBoeuf, Ph.D., author of *Imagineering,* suggests: Simply sit down and do nothing the next time you're having trouble getting started on something. The sheer boredom is likely to kick you into gear.

For more information, consult *The Now Habit: A Strategic Program for Overcoming Procrastination and Enjoying Guilt-Free Play* by Dr. Fiore.

The Serenity Prayer ▶ Yes, some stress is inevitable and even necessary for survival. Nothing ventured, after all, nothing gained. But there's a fine line between challenging ourselves and simply frustrating ourselves by attempting the impossible. And that's where the following "serenity prayer" can come in handy, says stress expert and best-selling author Joan Borysenko, Ph.D. It goes something like this: "Give me the serenity to accept the things that I cannot change, the courage to change the things that I can, and the wisdom to know the difference."

Get the point? Stress for a lot of us is the result of biting off more than we can chew and refusing to let go.

Meditation

Forget the gurus searching for nirvana. Meditation is for anyone looking for a little more peace here on earth. It involves simply taking a few quiet moments to focus your attention on a specific thought, word, sound, or bodily sensation, such as breathing. The goal is not immediate relaxation. Rather, meditation helps settle the mind so it can process thoughts calmly, in an organized way, throughout the day.

How often do you find your mind racing around in a dozen directions? Maybe you've even quipped, "I'm losing my mind." This isn't unusual. "People basically do live 'out of their minds' a lot of the time," explains Jon Kabat–Zinn, Ph.D., director of the stress reduction and relaxation program at the University of Massachusetts Medical Center. "Meditation can help us get back in control by forcing us to be present in the moment and observing our thought processes.

"That's what meditation comes down to," Dr. Kabat–Zinn says. "Paying attention, on purpose, in the present moment.

"It's a shock to many people the first time they meditate. They find they can't focus their attention on one breath without their mind jumping around," he explains. "Ironically, however, once you become aware of the chaos, your mind starts to calm down."

It's important to remember that when you notice your mind wandering during meditation, you shouldn't judge it; that creates stress. Just gently pull yourself back

261

to the present moment by redirecting your attention to the word or thought you're meditating on.

To ensure success, stress-management experts agree, you must come to meditation with an openness to explore the method fully (not just go through the motions) and a commitment to practice it on a regular basis. Only then can you realize its full potential.

Here are some specific meditation techniques.

Mindfulness Meditation ▶ There's nothing more powerful or accessible to anchor you in the moment than your breathing, says Dr. Kabat–Zinn. Sit comfortably, close your eyes, and focus on your breath for 5 minutes. Don't try to change or control it. Just watch it go in and out. Ride the waves of your breathing. Your mind will wander. That's okay. When it happens, bring your thoughts back to your breathing.

Dr. Kabat–Zinn calls this technique mindfulness meditation. Its advantage over other forms of meditation is that it's effective in small doses. Take a few seconds every hour or 5 minutes periodically throughout the day to practice mindfulness. Think of it as a breath of fresh mental air. The focusing on your breathing, even if it's only for a few seconds, can give the body subtle cues to relax that it wouldn't otherwise receive, Dr. Kabat–Zinn says. It also can give the brain a quick perk-up.

For more information on mindfulness, consult *Full Catastrophe Living: Using the Wisdom of Your Body and Mind to Face Stress, Pain and Illness* by Dr. Kabat–Zinn. Dr. Kabat–Zinn also offers audiocassette tapes on mindfulness. For more information, write to Stress Reduction Tapes, P.O. Box 547, Lexington, MA 02173.

The Relaxation Response ▶ Popularized by Harvard Medical School professor Herbert Benson, M.D., the Relaxation Response uses meditation to combat stress and revitalize the mind. It begins with selecting a word (such as *peace* or *one*) or a short prayer or meaningful phrase.

To give it a try: Sit in a comfortable position. Close your eyes and relax your muscles. Now, breathe slowly and naturally. On the exhale, repeat your word or phrase.

Try to disregard outside thoughts, but remain relaxed and passive if they do intrude. Continue the technique for 10 to 20 minutes once or twice daily.

For more information on the Relaxation Response, see *Your Maximum Mind* by Dr. Benson and William Proctor.

Transcendental Meditation ▶ Another meditative discipline, Transcendental Meditation (TM), has proved its stress-reducing effectiveness through years of scientific scrutiny. Yet it remains cloaked in mystery and misunderstanding even today. "It's not a philosophy or religion but an actual technique," says Gary Korf, a TM instructor and administrator with the World Plan Executive Council, the TM organization. "It comes from a long tradition that's been passed down from teacher to student."

What sets TM apart from the other meditation techniques listed here is that you can't learn it by reading a book or listening to a tape. You must take a seven-step course, including two lectures and four consecutive days of personal 2-hour instruction by a qualified TM teacher.

During the course, you are presented with a secret mantra (a certain sound to meditate on) chosen just for you. Mantras have no meaning to the meditator, but TM instructors say the sound quality is conducive to the meditation process.

Instructors also maintain that TM is effortless because it utilizes the natural tendency of the mind. "If you're sitting in a library trying to read a book and there's an interesting conversation on the other side of the shelf, you may read the page six times before you realize you haven't read a word. Our attention naturally tends to go to that which is more charming. The TM technique makes use of that," says Korf.

Intrigued? Bear in mind that course fees run about

$400 for an adult, $600 for a family, or $200 for a retired person. Once learned, TM should be practiced for 20 minutes twice a day.

For more information, check under Transcendental Meditation in the Yellow Pages, or write to TM Executive Council, 5000 14th Street NW, Washington, DC 20011. To learn more about the technique and program, consult *Maharishi Mahesh Yogi's TM* by Robert Roth.

Meditation Walking ▶ Walk away from stress? Exactly. The exercise alone helps relieve tension. And, when combined with meditation, it becomes an especially powerful tool in stress management.

But how is it possible to become lost in your thoughts while keeping your feet firmly on the path? Simply by going cheerfully (with a half-smile) and by establishing a relaxing rhythm between your breathing and your steps, says Thich Nhat Hanh in his book *A Guide to Walking Meditation*.

"Walk more slowly than you usually do, but not too slowly, while breathing normally. Do not try to control your breathing. Walk along in this way for a few minutes. Then notice how many steps you take as your lungs fill and how many steps you take as they empty. In this way, your attention includes both breath and steps. You are mindful of both. The link is the counting."

And as you walk, leave your stressful world behind. "To do this," says Hanh, "you have to learn to let go—let go of your sorrows, let go of your worries. That is the secret of walking meditation."

For more information, consult Hanh's book. To order send $6.95 plus $2.50 for postage and handling to Fellowship of Reconciliation, P.O. Box 271, Nyack, NY 10960.

Soul Pursuits

A woman bothered by stress-related headaches finds relief by purchasing clothing for needy children. A business executive finds peace with every turn of the shovel as he prepares for a second planting of string beans after a chaotic day at the office. A beleaguered housewife returns home refreshed and frisky after a quick three-day weekend in the mountains. Is there a common theme here?

Yes. These people are fighting stress by lifting their spirits and nourishing their souls. They're giving more perspective and meaning to their lives by taking time to see and experience the bigger picture.

Many of us go through a lot of unnecessary stress simply by failing to get off our treadmills often enough, the experts say. We get ourselves into ruts that can leave us feeling isolated, depressed, tired, and trapped.

But it doesn't have to be that way. Simply by expanding our experiences, we can enlarge our world. And by enlarging our world, we give life's daily snags less importance. We've got to take off our blinders, the experts say, and learn that straight ahead is not the only way to look. Peace of mind is better found by looking all around. Read on and see how.

Gardening ▶ More lurks out amidst the lettuce leaves than nutrition for the body: There's also nourishment for the soul. "Gardening is a natural, stress-releasing activity without the contrivance and inconvenience of working out at a health club," says Bryant Stamford, Ph.D., a professor of allied health at the University of Louisville, and coauthor of *Fitness without Exercise*.

Stress-management expert Emmett Miller, M.D., agrees. "Gardening takes our mind off the unsolvable problems we confront every day. It gives us work to do where we can see progress from minute to minute." And from month to month, as we see the fruits of our labors grow. Don't think that growing vegetables is the only way to destress, however. Gardens of flowers, herbs, fruit trees, or rocks can be equally soothing retreats.

Giving ▶ Not only is it more noble to give than to receive, it may also be healthier.

When we help others on a personal basis, we help ourselves by reducing stress. It draws our attention away from ourselves, and with the attention goes anxiety, says Alan Lucks of the Institute for the Advancement of Health in New York. Charitable behavior also seems to diminish feelings of isolation and loneliness, which sometimes can produce stress.

Simply exercising one's checkbook, though, may not be enough to produce these dividends. Direct contact seems to be a necessary part of the process. "It's also a good idea for people to get involved with a cause they really care about," says Lucks. "Otherwise there may be a feeling of resentment in the giving, which can reduce its stress-reducing benefits. Keeping involved on a regular basis also seems to be important—doing something weekly, for example."

For more information on the power of giving, watch for Lucks's book *Beyond Self*.

Sex ▶ Yes, sex involves arousal, but it can also—if it's good—promote profound relaxation, says Joshua Golden, M.D., director of the human sexuality program at UCLA. Most people, after all, go to sleep following a good frolic, so it's got to be doing something right.

Then, too, there are the emotional benefits of a healthy sexual relationship—you're establishing the security of a meaningful bond with another person, Dr. Golden says. Add the self-esteem that a good sex life can help nourish and you've got a stress buster with few equals. What other activity can do so much, not just for you but for someone else?

It's something to think about the next time you're tempted to turn on the television instead of your mate.

For more information on what it takes to maintain a healthy sex life, ask your family physician, local medical center, or county medical society to refer you to an appropriate professional. Or send a self-addressed stamped envelope to the American Association of Sex Educators, Counselors and Therapists (AA-SECT) for a free directory of certified sex educators, counselors, and therapists in your state. Their address is 435 North Michigan Avenue, Suite 1717, Chicago, IL 60611.

Vacations ▶ The vacation—the Rolls-Royce of stress reduction, right?

Careful. Yes, vacations can vanquish stress but they can also evoke it, says Richard J. Gitelson, Ph.D., of the Department of Leisure Studies at Pennsylvania State University. Danger lies in the vacation that's poorly planned and, hence, rife with decisions regarding meals and lodging that need to be made on the spot. Also stressful is the whirlwind vacation that tries to do too much.

The best vacation strikes a balance between being exciting and fun but also being relaxing, Dr. Gitelson says. You want a sense of adventure, but you don't want to be pulling your hair out to get it. This is why tours are becoming more and more popular, Dr. Gitelson says. The worrisome details are eliminated, but not the sense of wonder.

Also growing in popularity are shorter vacations, Dr. Gitelson says—two- to three-day outings rather than two-week marathons. Vacations dedicated to stress reduction and health improvement specifically also are gaining in favor.

Keeping a Journal ▶ Not only is the pen mightier than the sword, it also can be mightier than the army of anxieties that keep us captive to stress. "Writing is a great way of unburdening ourselves," says James Pennebaker, Ph.D., author of *Opening Up: The Healing Powers of Confiding in Others*. "It's a way of putting our problems into a more manageable form that can make them more understandable and perhaps even a little easier to solve."

Dr. Pennebaker has done studies with college students showing that those who participated in writing sessions reduced their blood pressure and boosted their immune system. He offers these tips.

Choose a place that's private and peaceful. Set a time limit for each session—20 to 30 minutes should do it. Write for the entire time, even if you find you're repeating yourself. As specifically as possible, write about what's troubling you, not just day-to-day events. Write with the

267

assurance that your thoughts need never be discovered by others, and be honest accordingly. Don't feel compelled to write every day (too much writing can be a substitute for action, Dr. Pennebaker says). For more information, see Dr. Pennebaker's book.

Antistress Breathing

We take breathing for granted. And why not? We've been doing it since the moment we were born. But doing is one thing, perfecting is another. Rapid, shallow breathing is often brought on by stress. And shallow breathing can fan the flames of stress, exacerbating feelings of anxiety and even causing panic attacks in some people. But proper breathing can blow stress away.

"Breathing is unique in that it's the only involuntary activity of the body over which we have conscious control," says Dr. Borysenko. "This provides a unique opportunity to take direct control over a basic physiological function that in turn slows the heartbeat, decreases the release of adrenaline, and creates harmony among the body systems."

The following three techniques are geared to helping you tap that source of calm.

Exhalation Breathing ▶ What deep breathing does, exhalation breathing tries to do even better: slow the quick and shallow breaths that are a stress trademark. "Rapid breathing causes problems by ridding the blood of too much carbon dioxide," explains Martin Pierce, director of the Atlanta-based Pierce Program, which specializes in stress reduction for professionals. Exhalation breathing puts on the brakes. Here's how to do it.

■ Lie down with your arms near your sides.

■ Begin to inhale, raising your arms (elbows bent) toward the ceiling as you do. Take them all the way over your head to the floor, if comfortable, by the time your inhalation is complete.

■ Reverse the procedure, focusing on a very slow,

smooth, and even exhalation as you slowly return your arms to your sides.

■ After several times, continue breathing in this way without moving your arms. Try to make the exhalations longer, but inhalations can be whatever speed is comfortable.

You can use this technique to help you relax on a daily basis, or you can employ it in a reduced form (without actually lying down or using the arm movements) to help you relax in the actual heat of battle.

Deep (Abdominal) Breathing ▶ "Deep breathing is one of the simplest yet most effective stress management techniques there is," says Dean Ornish, M.D., author of *Dr. Dean Ornish's Program for Reversing Heart Disease.* "You can do it anywhere, any time, and it becomes even more effective with practice." How does deep breathing work?

It infuses the blood with extra oxygen but also causes the body to release endorphins, which are natural tranquilizing hormones. To enjoy the benefits of deep breathing, however, you have to do it from the abdomen, not just the chest. This allows the lower lobes of the lungs (which accept oxygen best) to become more involved in the breathing process. Here's how to do it.

■ Slowly inhale through your nose, expanding your abdomen before allowing air to fill your chest.

■ Slowly reverse the process as you exhale.

Take a few minutes each day to practice this technique.

Qigong Breathing ▶ The Chinese art of Qigong is believed to reduce stress, as well as revitalize the body. It wasn't founded on scientific research, but the Chinese have used it avidly for a long time.

Qigong is done in combination with exercises that enhance or facilitate its breathing techniques. "In China it has been said that there are over 4,000 styles of Qigong exercises," says Qigong master Effie Chow, Ph.D., of the East-West Academy of Healing Arts, in San Francisco. But for the purposes of combating stress, her clients like this "heavenly stretch" the best.

■ With no music and no distraction, stand up straight with your feet together and your eyes straight forward and exhale.

■ Now slowly inhale and stretch your arms as high up over your head as you can. Lift up onto your toes, feeling the stretch all the way down to your ankles. "Imagine a silver thread running up through your spine and pulling you upward," Dr. Chow says.

■ Continue taking in small bits of air as you make this stretch.

■ At the pinnacle, begin exhaling slowly, letting your arms float back down to your sides as you do. Flex your wrists, pushing your palms downward.

Dr. Chow recommends a sequence of eight of these stretches daily to increase your resiliency to stress. To learn more Qigong exercises, Dr. Chow recommends that you find a qualified instructor.

For more information, write to the Qigong Institute, East-West Academy of Healing Arts, 450 Sutter Street, Suite 916, San Francisco, CA 94108.

Soothing Sights and Sounds

Have you ever had a beautiful sunset suddenly fill you with a sense of awe? For a brief but wonderful moment you're overwhelmed, and you suddenly forget your worldly woes. Or maybe you've had a similar experience with a great piece of music, the scent of a rose bush in bloom, or the pleasing flavors of a great meal.

What soothes the senses tends to calm the mind. Pleasure in its most natural forms can satisfy us so deeply that our stress gets pushed aside momentarily.

270

Music ▶ Some experts theorize it's the rhythm, some say it's the "tonal atmospheres" created by music, others say it's just feeling comfortable with whatever you like. And although it's not scientifically proven, few people would disagree that music can work soothing magic. Here are some music-centered techniques to try.

■ Heartfelt rhythm. The idea here is to listen to music that has a tempo slightly slower than your heart rate, says Kansas City music therapist Janalea Hoffman. This not only encourages the heart to slow down to keep in sync, but it can momentarily lower blood pressure as well. "The average heart beats 60 to 68 times per minute, so I write music with 50 to 60 beats per minute," she says.

This is considerably slower than most popular music being written today, so you'll have to do some shopping around to get tunes that fit the bill. Some classical suggestions: Bach's *Brandenburg Concerto No. 4,* 2nd movement, Bach's *Orchestral Suite No. 2* ("Saraband"), Holst's *The Planets* ("Venus"), Ravel's *Mother Goose Suite,* 1st movement.

■ Toning out. Music relaxes us by turning us loose, not by taking us by the hand, says composer and psychologist Steven Halpern, Ph.D., author of *Sound Health.* Nor is rhythm the only element to be considered. Melody, too, can be too bullish. So what you get from Halpern and the other New Age composers are not so much songs as tonal landscapes, musical moods with very little melody and equally little beat. Here are some of Dr. Halpern's top picks if you'd like to give the New Age route a try: *Silk Road* by Kitaro, *Spectrum Suite* by Steven Halpern, *Inside* by Paul Horn, *Valley of the Birds* by Emerald Web, *Autumn* by George Winston. Or for a catalog of other New Age tunes, write for Alcazar's New Music Collection, P.O. Box 429, Waterbury, VT 05676. Or call toll-free (800) 541-9904.

■ Finding your comfort tones. If Aerosmith helps you relax more than Debussy, so be it. That's the thinking of Radford University director of music therapy Joseph Scartelli, Ph.D. "Sitting down and forcing yourself to listen to relaxation music that you don't like may create stress, not alleviate it," he says.

271

Wind Chimes ▶ Yes, you may cast your stress to the wind if you've got the right set of chimes, says Dr. Halpern. The random melodic "music" created by wind chimes can create a very soothing environment—if that's your cup of tea. But it's important to choose chimes that are in tune with one another so that harmony is created rather than mere noise, Dr. Halpern says. The most soothing sounds of all are produced by aluminum or copper tubular chimes measuring 12 to 18 inches in length, he contends.

For more information or a free catalog of seven different precision-tuned models, write or call Woodstock Chimes, Route 1, Box 381A, West Hurley, NY 12491; (800) 422-4463.

Glimpses of Nature ▶ What the ears can do, the eyes may do as well—at least in the realm of stress lessening. "Anything that holds your attention so that you're looking and listening instead of thinking and worrying can reduce stress," says University of Pennsylvania psychiatrist Aaron Katcher, M.D. Just watching a campfire or fireplace, going bird-watching, taking a walk in the park, or watching fish in an aquarium can do it. Dr. Katcher says that doing any of these kinds of activities for 15 minutes or so twice a day can have measurable stress-lowering effects.

If you'd really like to give your mind a breath of fresh air, expand your horizons, says stress expert Emmett Miller, M.D., author of *Software for the Mind*. Long-distance views of natural surroundings may be our best eye-pleasers of all because they inspire us with feelings of openness and hope.

Take walks outside whenever possible. Or simply imagine yourself in some breathtakingly open environment, Dr. Miller says. Put yourself on a mountaintop in the Swiss Alps at sunrise. "If you really concentrate on that image, you'll feel a sense of relief," he says.

If you just can't get out and you're not good at imagining, you might try listening to recordings of nature sounds. They're available at record stores. Some tapes, such as "Peaceful Evening" and "Misty Forest Morning" by Steve and David Gordon, combine instrumentals with nature sounds. Order these from Sequoia Records, Dept. SQR, Box 280, Topanga, CA 90290; (800) 824-4000, ext. 939.

Another option, nature videotapes, may suit you even better. One produced by Dr. Miller, for example, takes you on a journey from a gentle forest glen to the wide expanse of the ocean. This video and others by Dr. Miller can be ordered through Source Cassettes, Inc., at (800) 52-TAPES. Nature videos can also be found in specialty bookstores or video-rental stores.

The Meditation Garden ▶ Just a little bit of nature can go a long way, it seems. That's been the theory behind the meditation garden for centuries. Meditation gardens, or Zen gardens, originated in Japan, and they're just what their name implies: places for peaceful reflection.

A meditation garden asks for your imagination more than your Rototiller. The most famous, Ryoan-ji in Kyoto, Japan, is nothing more than a rectangle of sand with 15 carefully placed stones and a little dark moss.

The idea is to sit and gaze reverently upon the garden's simple features, which become metaphors for nature. To the Japanese, for example, a rock might come to represent a towering, majestic mountain; an area of sand or gravel raked into smooth and winding patterns becomes a river meandering through a valley. However small, meditation gardens should convey a sense of expansiveness and peace.

For more information on creating your own meditation garden, consult *Theme Gardens* by Barbara Damrosch.

Relaxation Training

There are times when relaxation comes naturally. But often, when you're under a lot of tension and need it most, you've got to work at it. Training yourself to relax—

mentally and physically—is the subject of the following techniques.

Guided Imagery ▶ When you employ guided imagery (also called directed visualization), you can use the mind's eye to help dissolve stress. By seeing pictures of relaxing situations in our minds, we can produce relaxing physiological changes in our bodies—momentarily lowering blood pressure and slowing heart rate, for example.

In his book *Healing Visualizations,* Gerald Epstein, M.D., offers this exercise for reducing anxiety: "Close your eyes and exhale three times. Imagine yourself at the ocean under a clear blue sky with your anxiety inside you like a stone. Let the wind and water erode the stone, washing and blowing it away. Know that when the stone is gone, your anxiety will be gone as well. The mind's eye also can help us make changes in our behavior that may be responsible for our stress in the first place. "

"By forming an image, a person makes a clear mental statement of what he or she wants to happen," write O. Carl Simonton, M.D., and Stephanie Matthews-Simonton in *Getting Well Again.* "As a result of positive expectation, the person begins to act in ways consistent with achieving the desired result."

Progressive Relaxation ▶ Developed by University of Chicago researcher Edmund Jacobson in the 1930s, progressive relaxation employs the mind in working to overcome tense muscles. Here's how to give it a try.

Lie down or sit in a comfortable chair in a quiet setting, close your eyes, and begin by making tight fists with your hands. Hold for 5 seconds, then relax, paying close attention to the draining of tension. Do this three times, noting the contrast between tension and relaxation. Do the same sequence throughout your body's various muscle groups: arms, forehead, mouth, shoulders, chest, abdomen, back, hips and thighs, lower legs, and feet. Try to limit each flex to the muscle group. Concentrate on the pleasurable feeling of release as you let the flex go.

At first it may take you 20 minutes or more to go

through the routine. But once you get proficient at this exercise, you can use as needed and complete the routine in 5 minutes.

Biofeedback ▶ Biofeedback is a system of learning to relax with the help of electronic monitoring devices that give you a report (feedback) on how your body reacts when stress strikes. By observing these body responses, you can then put your mind to work to alter them in a healthier direction.

Some biofeedback units measure stress by measuring perspiration (released in response to stress). They emit tones that range in pitch according to perspiration production. By attending to the tonal changes and applying relaxation, you may learn to control specific stress responses. But before dashing off to buy a biofeedback machine, it's important to first consult with a professional counselor to find out which body signs might be best for you to monitor. "Everyone has a different physiologic profile of stress symptoms," says Lynn Becker, Ed.D., a psychologist at the Veterans Administration Medical Center in Battle Creek, Michigan.

For more information on biofeedback or a list of certified practitioners in your area, write the Biofeedback Certification Institute of America (BCIA), 10200 West 44th Avenue, #304, Wheat Ridge, CO 80033; please enclose a self-addressed, stamped envelope.

Antistress Baths

As noted at the beginning of this chapter, the war against stress can be waged in two ways: You can get at its causes or you can simply treat its symptoms. Cause control is the better and more lasting approach, of course, but that doesn't mean that symptom soothing doesn't also have value. By soothing our symptoms of stress, in fact, we improve our chances of getting in the frame of mind it may take to understand and do something about its causes. So consider the following information with that in mind.

■

The Evening Soak ▶ "It's my daily oasis," says one working mother. "I get in that tub and my troubles melt." That may sound poetic, but it has some science on its side. Warm baths work by relaxing the muscles but also perhaps by slightly heating the brain, which can be calming, experts say. Notice the word *warm*, however. If water is too hot it can shock the system, causing muscles to constrict. Water between 100° and 102°F (that's comfortably warm to the touch) is best. Soak for no more than 15 minutes.

Steam Baths and Saunas ▶ And what about scorching steam baths and saunas for washing away life's woes? They may work if you're willing to undergo the discomfort, says Edward R. Eichner, M.D., University of Oklahoma Health Sciences Center. As David I. Abramson writes in the *Journal of the American Medical Association*, with tongue firmly planted in cheek, the calming effects of a steam bath or sauna might "be compared with the great feeling of relief experienced by the patient who has been suffering from severe pain and suddenly finds that he has become free of symptoms."

If that sort of approach to relief sounds like your style, you might give the hot stuff a try. Check first with your doctor, however, as steam baths and saunas can put quite a strain on the cardiovascular system.

Tub Relaxation ▶ You can mellow out even more from a bath if you combine it with some progressive relaxation, says Carole B. Lewis, Ph.D., of George Washington University and the University of Pittsburgh. Let your hand float gently on the water, then allow that feeling of relaxation to flow to your elbow, then to your upper arm and shoulder, and finally to your head. Let the soothing sensation flow to any area of your body that might feel tense.

Flotation Tanks ▶ Take a large bathtub, fill it with warm water and lots of Epsom salts to increase buoyancy, then encase it in a sealed, soundproof container—and you've got what some are calling nirvana in a box. The profound silence and elimination of almost all external stimuli offers the stress-busting ultimate, says Peter Suedfeld, Ph.D., of the University of British Columbia. Theories vary on how they work, Dr. Suedfeld says.

For more information, check your local Yellow Pages under "Flotation," "Isolation Tanks," or just "Tanks," if you're interested in giving the experience a try. Or contact the Flotation Tank Association at P.O. Box 1396, Grass Valley, CA 95945; cost is $15 to $50 per 45- to 60-minute float.

Bath Herbals ▶ To help make that soothing plunge even more celestial, try buoying your bath with some fragrance. Numerous commercial preparations are available, but you can also concoct your own by making a "tea" from your favorite herbs or flowers. Just add 1 quart of boiling water to 1 cup of leaves or flower buds. Allow to cool, strain the liquid, and add it to your bath water.

Body Destressors

Stress may start in the mind, but it winds up in the body. Muscles tighten. Nerves become hypersensitive to pain. This makes you irritable. Which makes the stress in your life even tougher to handle. Which makes you even more irritable. Which makes your pain worse . . .

At some point the escalating cycle has to be broken. And if you can't do it mentally, perhaps you can do it physically. That's the theory behind the following stress busters that seek to grab the physical symptoms of stress by the horns.

Massage ▶ When faced with stress our body often tightens, causing pain. For some individuals, massage can help relieve this muscle tension and bring about a sense of relaxation.

Shiatsu is a form of massage based on Chinese medicine that has been recorded since 200 B.C. According to Cindy Banker, president of the American Shiatsu Association, "In Shiatsu massage, pressure is applied to specific energetic pathways in the body, freeing up tension. There's one such area located on the wrist, for example, where blockage can reflect feelings of anxiety," she claims. "It's approximately two thumb widths from the bottom of your palm. Press on it as you take a deep breath followed by a long, slow exhalation. You may feel some relief right away."

A full Shiatsu treatment strategically performs similar proddings all over the body, finding areas of tightness and working them out. If you'd like to try a Shiatsu treatment, contact the American Shiatsu Association at P.O. Box 718, Jamaica Plain, MA 02130; (617) 236-5867. They can refer you to a certified practitioner in your area. (If you write, include $1 to cover postage for the ASA directory they'll send.) And, of course, there are many other types of massage, all of which can be great destressors. To find out where to experience these other types firsthand, call or write to the American Massage Therapy Association at 1130 West North Shore, Chicago, IL 60626; (312) 761-AMTA. They can refer you to a massage therapist in your area. If you and your spouse or a friend would like to learn massage to help each other let go of stress, you may find the video "Massage for Health" helpful. It comes with a 40-page book and a free bottle of massage oil. Call toll-free to Healing Arts Home Video, (800) 722-7347.

Yoga ▶ Through combinations of movement, breathing awareness, and relaxation techniques, yoga can reduce stress in three ways, says Linda Cogozzo, managing editor of *Yoga Journal*. It gives you time out to focus on yourself, which helps set the stage for stress reduction. It improves breathing, muscle tone, and posture, which can help you combat stress physically.

And it "helps you get in touch with how you're really feeling," Cogozzo says.

"When you can identify your problems, they lose some of their hold on you. Yoga helps you do that by cultivating your ability to be aware of yourself physically and emotionally."

Yoga also can help you carry yourself in a way that can combat stress by giving you a greater sense of self-esteem. "Shoulders relaxed, chest lifted, legs strong. Holding your body in this position, called Mountain Pose, gives a message to your mind about what it's like to feel confident," says Cogozzo. The good posture that yoga teaches can also combat low back pain, which can be a great source and cause of stress.

For a good introduction to yoga, Cogozzo recommends "Yoga for Beginners," a 75-minute video accompanied by a 52-page instructional book. She also advises working with a qualified instructor. "Yoga is something that needs to be learned correctly and practiced regularly in order to produce optimum results. Even if you do just one pose a day, it's important to keep the thread going." For a copy of the video, call Healing Arts Home Video at (800) 722-7347.

Body Stretching ▶ Is it stretching the point to suggest a limber body can lead to a limber mind, more resilient to the assaults of stress?

No, says Dr. Ornish. "Stretching can help you feel more peaceful and relaxed. Just as your mind affects your body, so can your body affect your mind."

There are right and wrong ways to attempt this loosening up, however, he says. First and foremost is to forget the creed of "no pain, no gain." Pain defeats the purpose of stretching by causing muscles to tighten rather than relax. So never bounce when you stretch. Here are some other stretching tips Dr. Ornish says can make stretching a stress breaker rather than a stress maker.

■ Think about the areas being stretched. Imagine the tension leaving them as you gently take them to their comfortable limit.

■ Move slowly and fluidly.

■ Exhale into the stretch; inhale on the release. Breathe deeply and slowly and always through the nose. Never hold your breath during a stretch.

■ Wear loose, comfortable clothing.

279

- Stretch with eyes closed for better awareness of body responses.

- Wait several hours after eating before stretching. Physical movement diverts blood from the digestive system.

- Enjoy the process; don't worry about the result.

That being said, here are some specific stretches to relieve stiff muscles.

- Sit up straight. Inhale. Exhale as you let gravity slowly pull your head down to your chest. Feel the gentle stretch to the back of your neck and shoulders. Now inhale as you slowly roll your right ear to your right shoulder, lifting your chin gently upward. Exhale as you drop your chin to your chest. Repeat to the left.

- Next, drop your arms to your sides. Push both shoulders forward. Slowly raise them toward your ears and circle them back and downward to the starting point. Do this slowly two or three times, then switch directions.

- Stand with your feet shoulder-width apart. Gently swing your arms from side to side, letting them flop. At the same time, allow your hips and torso to rotate comfortably.

Walking ▶ Yes, you can simply step away from stress—temporarily, at least—with what may be our oldest stress reducer of all, the walk. Studies by California State University psychologist Robert Thayer, Ph.D., have shown significant reductions in tension after walks lasting only several minutes.

Better yet, the walks left people feeling energized in addition to feeling calm—the best of both worlds! Another study by Florida's State Department of Health and Rehabilitative Services found that participants in an eight-week walking program were able to reduce the stress they felt at work by 30 percent.

How does walking work?

Several factors are probably at play, researchers say.

Walking can provide a needed escape, but it also may increase the body's production of the mood-elevating brain chemicals called endorphins. It also may help us feel better about ourselves if we do it to the point of losing body fat or improving physical fitness. A poor self-image, after all, can add an element of stress to virtually everything we do.

Jaw Stretching ▶ Bothered by pain or stiffness in the jaw area? Certainly there can be many causes. But it's possible you may be part of the 22 percent of the population known as jaw clenchers, which means you unconsciously clench your jaws tightly and put undue strain on jaw muscles. You may even be grinding your teeth in addition to clenching, which can really give jaw muscles a tough time. Dentists know that these habits occur most commonly in highly stressed people, and they think that stress may be a cause (although it could possibly be an effect).

If you have this problem, you may help relieve the resulting pain and stiffness simply by stretching your jaw muscles, says New York dentist, John Dodes, D.D.S. The exercises, developed at Columbia University, keep the muscles and ligaments of the jaw area limber. Slowly open your mouth as widely as you comfortably can—ten times. Now make a fist, put it beneath your chin, and open your mouth against some mild resistance from your fist—three times.

Repeating this sequence 12 or so times a day will not cure you of your jaw-clenching habit. But it may help eliminate the pain caused by muscle cramps and spasms, Dr. Dodes says.

The Instant-Calming Sequence ▶ Most stress-reduction methods concentrate on unraveling the knots of stress after they've been securely tied, but not so with the instant-calming sequence (ICS), says Robert K. Cooper, Ph.D., president of Advanced Excellence Systems in Bemidji, Minnesota. The ICS method, once learned, may neutralize the potentially negative effects of a stressful situation in "less than 1 second," he claims.

And the instant-calming sequence can be used anytime and anywhere: to help you handle unexpected bad news, to help you make critical decisions, to keep you calm in the face of an argument, to help you relax in traffic jams, even to help you ward off nagging feelings of worry or guilt.

Here's how to do it.

■ Train yourself to continue breathing normally. "Most of us halt our breathing for several seconds or more during the first moments of a stressful situation," Dr. Cooper says. This reduces oxygen to the brain and can push us toward feelings such as anxiety, panic, anger, frustration, and loss of control.

■ Keep your facial expression positive. Some scientists speculate that a positive expression, no matter what your mental state, may increase blood flow to the brain and transmit nerve impulses to a key emotional center there that can help prevent feelings of distress and keep you in better control of challenging or difficult situations. "Even the slightest smile may help prevent the nervous system from overreacting to negative stress," Dr. Cooper says.

■ Keep good upright posture. Many of us collapse into a slouching position when hit with a stressful situation, Dr. Cooper says. This not only restricts breathing and reduces blood flow to the brain, it also adds needless muscle tension and can magnify feelings of helplessness. "Keep your posture buoyant when stress strikes," Dr. Cooper says.

■ Take a quick tension inventory. With one fast mental sweep, try to notice any area of your body that may be tightening—from your scalp clear down to your toes—and imagine the tension being released as if standing under a soothing waterfall.

■ Maintain mental calm and clarity. Too often, when faced with a stressful situation, we react emotionally, blaming ourselves or others or bemoaning the hand we've been dealt. When we do this, however, we lose our ability to control the situation and improve the outcome. What's better? Simply acknowledge and accept what's happening. Then you will be much better prepared to choose a wiser response.

"That's the key to the ICS—learning to insert that calm, clear-mindedness in precisely the right place at the very beginning of each stress scene," says Dr. Cooper. With practice, you can train your mind to quickly seek positive solutions.

For further instruction on the ICS, consult Dr. Cooper's book *Health and Fitness Excellence.*

T'ai Chi Ch'uan ▶ T'ai chi is an ancient, gentle discipline of meditative exercises practiced by millions of Chinese. It consists of slow, flowing, dancelike motions.

"T'ai chi has emotional as well as physiological benefits," says Gene Strickland, an instructor with the New Center for Holistic Health Education and Research in Manhasset, New York. "It forces you to focus on your body rather than your problems. It also teaches proper posture and breathing."

Practicing this calming exercise takes some study: A short form of t'ai chi includes about 54 different postures (bearing names such as Grasp Sparrow's Tail and Snake Creeps Down) and takes about 15 minutes to perform.

To learn t'ai chi, which can take years to fully master, you should be trained by a qualified instructor.

For more information, check with organizations offering continuing education courses or under martial arts or t'ai chi in the Yellow Pages. An excellent book on t'ai chi is *Tao and T'ai Chi Kung* by Robert C. Sohn, Ph.D.

Is Your Relationship Fit?   33

By Harold Bloomfield, M.D., Sirah Vettese,
Ph.D., and Robert Kory

Can you and your mate or lover freely reveal to each
other who you really are and what you really want—good
and bad, strengths and weaknesses, hopes and fears,
successes and failures?

For many couples, the answer is at best a qualified
yes, but for others it is no. Most people are afraid to let
others, even a lover, know what they really feel about
important personal issues. Lack of self-confidence, hidden
resentments, painful memories, and secret desires are
universal, but few couples know how to help each other
accept and resolve these powerful but hidden feelings.

Most couples spend less than 30 minutes per week
sharing their most intimate feelings. No wonder relationships go stale. Rather than explore their feelings, many
people assume they know how the other partner feels
when in reality they are each afraid to ask. For love to
remain exciting and vibrant, intense and deeply honest,
communication of feelings is vital.

To begin, an assessment of fears that stand in the
way of heart-to-heart communication is helpful. For some
people, a fear of rejection is a primary inhibition. Almost
everyone harbors some anxiety that if a lover really knew
everything, rejection might be the result. Other people
fear their own anger. They resist exposing their deepest
feelings because they sense a rage that could lead to
violence. Still others fear an encounter with their own
self-image. They fear that letting a lover know them will
be humiliating or lead them to feel inferior.

Those who desperately seek love and find it may
discover a new worry—the fear of losing that love and
once again being left to face life alone. The persistence of

such fears makes creating and sustaining a great love relationship difficult, if not impossible.

Withholding such feelings creates a burden on you and your relationship by undermining self-confidence and your ability to give and accept love. When two people hide their deepest feelings, the relationship is doomed to boredom and chronic frustration. Instead of making their needs clear, couples begin to manipulate, intimidate, or induce guilt in each other. Affairs and divorce often follow.

Defusing Fears

How do you overcome fears of self-disclosure that block heart-to-heart communication with your love partner? We have developed a series of love fitness workouts called "Heart Talks," based on the psychological principle that the best way to expand the capacity for love is to let go of fear. Heart Talks establish an emotional environment of care, safety, and trust, allowing both you and your lover to accept and enjoy the risk of self-disclosure, discover hidden parts of yourselves, and develop new emotional connections. Those who learn and practice Heart Talks report that these exercises are exciting, challenging, and often lots of fun.

Heart Talks involve much more than saccharine sentimentality. They are designed to help you discover the courage to be vulnerable, to divulge insecurities and pain, to endure conflict and struggles, and to share your dreams and hopes. Heart Talks instill the safety and trust necessary to do the psychological housecleaning that every intimate relationship requires. Even if your lover is uncooperative at first, the more self-disclosing you are, the more open and honest others will be around you. Talk from your heart and soon your lifemate will join you. Keep in mind, however, that although self-disclosure is essential to personal growth and intimacy, it is a process to be undertaken carefully. Total openness can impose an unrealistic standard upon love and mar-

285
∎

riage. To say that husband and wife should keep no secrets from one another and that complete honesty is always the best policy fails to recognize the human need for some zones of privacy.

If you don't feel comfortable sharing the sexual details of a past romance, there is no reason to feel as if you must. Also, there is no obligation to reveal a sexual fantasy or secret that you feel is just too personal to share even with your lifemate. Intimacy does not mean you have to tell your lover everything!

Self-disclosure must be done safely and in measures appropriate to the situation. There are some disclosures that may lead to disabling or even terminating a love relationship, rather than strengthening it.

We are not condoning affairs, which we see as an emotional escape valve that many resort to as a result of their lack of love fitness. What we are saying is that without a trained counselor in attendance, a confession of this nature may trigger consequences that neither partner anticipates.

The revelation of a one-night stand that would have no further consequence can actually lead to serious impairment or destruction of a relationship.

Heart Talks can be misused to analyze a relationship to its death. Some people enter a relationship with the false assumption that they must expose and analyze every facet of their lifemate's psyche. Heart Talks are never meant for playing armchair psychiatrist with your love partner. If you discuss each other's traits ad nauseum, you may drive each other crazy. When communication is usurped by endless confrontation, introspection, and psyche searching, it is appropriate to say to your lover, "Tell me less" rather than "Tell me more."

Almost any truth or value taken to an extreme becomes false. So too with the value of openness. Getting to know and be known by a lover is exciting and emotionally enriching. Angrily "letting it all hang out" can be unkind as well as unwise, however. Just as important to intimacy as openness are propriety and good taste.

There is no excuse for napalming your spouse's self-esteem.

One last caution: Heart Talks are not a cure for a relationship on the rocks. If you are in a marital crisis, or feel your relationship is poor or unstable, or that you or your partner will react negatively to intimate sharing, it is best to contact a trained mental health expert or marriage counselor to assist in safely exploring self-disclosure and dealing with the subsequent issues that may emerge.

The Ground Rules

The instructions for Heart Talk exercises are very simple, but strict adherence to a few rules is necessary to create the emotional safety and trust to make Heart Talks work. So before trying a Heart Talk, both of you should make the following agreements with each other (read these aloud before beginning your Heart Talks).

1. I promise never to interrupt you.

2. I promise not to withdraw emotionally or to leave physically; I will not reject you for anything you wish to share.

3. I will make it safe for you to express your most intimate feelings; I will stay open and vulnerable to you.

4. Nothing you say will be used against you or to provoke an argument later.

5. I will be responsible for my emotions, and I will not blame you for how I feel. If I do blame or complain, I will take immediate responsibility for doing so, and stop.

6. I will share the truth from my heart as caringly, honestly, and respectfully as I can.

7. I will love you unconditionally and use any block or conflict that may arise as a stimulus to more learning and greater love.

8. I will try not to manipulate, defend, or control what you communicate.

9. I commit to dealing with and working through any barriers that come up in our Heart Talks until there is resolution and we are once again open and loving with each other.

10. I agree that we can disagree. As we may not see eye to eye about all issues, we will each allow the other his/her feelings, understanding, and point of view.

11. I agree to finish each Heart Talk session with at least one embracing hug (remember, five hugs a day keeps the marriage counselor away) and a sincere "I love you."

Also, you need to create an appropriate environment for your Heart Talks. Disconnect the phone and take precautions against outside interruption. Until you learn to be "in close," it is important to set up a "proper distance." Use comfortable chairs placed 3 to 3½ feet apart, allowing for eye contact and enough "space" to be able to deal with any difficult feelings that may emerge.

Set a time limit at first—at least 30 minutes but not more than an hour per sitting. This will preempt the tendency to "feel like quitting" when resistances come up. Just as with a physical fitness program, three ½-hour sessions a week is the minimum necessary for love fitness, while a full 1-hour workout once every week or two will allow for even greater intimacy with your lifemate.

Exercises for Intimacy

The following exercises will launch you into Heart Talks, providing a framework for heart-to-heart communication. For each Heart Talk session, choose exercises from the appropriate level and take turns completing the incomplete sentences. (You should each complete the same sentences.) Each level will have you exploring a different degree of intimacy and personal privacy, ranging from the least-intimate discussions in Level 1 to the greatest in Level 4.

Level 1: Explorations

1. The three people in history I would most like to have as dinner guests in our home are . . .

2. The personal and professional goals I want to accomplish in the next year are . . . in the next five years are . . .

3. A one-month, all-expense-paid trip I would like to take anywhere in the world is . . .

4. The three people who have done the most to influence my values and thinking are . . .

5. How I feel about divorce is . . .

6. What I like best about my work and career is . . .

7. If I could have three magic wishes, I would wish for . . .

8. My feelings about being/becoming a parent are . . .

9. I would like to spend more of our time . . .

10. It would please me greatly if you were interested in . . .

11. What I have noticed recently about myself is . . .

12. Three objects, representing significant events in our life together, that I value most are . . .

Level 2: Feelings

1. The two biggest personal challenges I am facing in my life at present are . . .

2. What I am most worried/concerned about this week is . . .

3. An important change I would like to see in you is . . .

4. If I could change one thing about how I was raised, it would be . . .

5. Personal or work habits I would like to change in myself are . . .

6. The reasons I have the "better deal" in our relationship are . . .

7. The reasons you have the "better deal" in our relationship are . . .

8. Three specific things that make you a pleasure to live with are . . .

9. Three specific things that make you difficult to live with are . . .

10. What I am most afraid of is . . .

11. My greatest anxieties are . . .

12. An unforgettable evening with you would be . . .

13. An important change I want to see in myself is . . .

Level 3: Ambivalences

1. Parts of my body and appearance I dislike the most are . . .

2. Parts of my body and appearance I feel best about are . . .

3. The most self-destructive behavior pattern I notice in me is . . .

4. The most self-destructive behavior pattern I notice in you is . . .

5. The three things I like least about my life are . . .

6. The three things I like best about my life are . . .

7. The way I would feel more loved by you is . . .

8. The aspects of my personality I worry about or regard as weaknesses are . . .

9. The three most treasured memories of our love are . . .

10. I have or haven't felt hatred for someone in my family because . . .

11. The five greatest achievements of my life are . . .

12. The time that I last cried by myself was . . . because . . .

13. The thing that I have dreamed about doing for a long time but have not done as yet is . . .

14. If friends and family gave me the worst possible but honest feedback about me, they would say . . .

Level 4: Secrets

1. The three most dishonest, dishonorable things I have ever done are . . .

2. Sometimes when I feel sexually excited, I . . .

3. Faults and disabilities I have and don't like to acknowledge are . . .

4. I've been secretly resentful about . . .

5. Two specific things I don't want you to know about me are . . .

6. If I were to die within the next 24 hours, what I would most want to communicate to you is . . .

7. The specific events in my life that have been the most traumatic and emotionally painful are . . .

8. The last time I wanted to scream and yell at you was . . . because . . .

9. My biggest disappointments in life have been . . .

10. My darkest secret is . . .

Late-Night Heart Talks

Some couples prefer to engage in Heart Talks at the end of the day while in bed. Lifemates take turns completing at least one of the statements.

1. What worked in my relationship with you today is . . .

The purpose is to share specific feelings, events, and observations that contributed in a constructive way to the overall enhancement of the relationship. You may identify something positive that your lover said or did during the day. You might also acknowledge yourself for some contribution to the relationship, such as a new way of behaving or the correction of an emotional habit that caused problems.

Here is an example from one client: "I noticed that when I took a wrong turn on our way to the meeting last night, you did not criticize me as you would have in the past. I asked for your assistance and acknowledged that I was unsure of how to get there. I felt good about my willingness to acknowledge a mistake and appreciated your understanding."

2. What did not work for me in my relationship with you today is . . .

291
■

Again, the statements that follow may be descriptions of the events, conversations, and observations that the speaker perceived as problems in the relationship. As the speaker shares those feelings, the listener does not interrupt or comment, except to say, "Tell me more." The purpose of this exercise is to create an opportunity for regular feedback in the relationship. The more specific the statement, the more easily appropriate adjustments can be made.

3. What worked in my relationship with me today is . . .

This exercise allows you to acknowledge and reinforce desirable habits and achievements. Here is another example from a client: "Although I felt tired at the end of the day, I took the time to walk on the beach and get my exercise. I felt great afterward, and I am glad that I took the time in spite of fatigue."

4. What did not work in my relationship with me today is . . .

This exercise is intended to assist lovers in acknowledging and encouraging their respective personal growth. For example, one client noted, "I was really a jerk for not being more assertive in today's presentation to a new customer. I need to improve my sales skills in this business." By inviting your lover to understand what changes you are trying to make in your own life and career, you give your lover an opportunity to understand your weaknesses and to help you develop new strengths. Such mutual disclosure allows you and your lover to better understand each other's personal struggles and feel supported.

These late-night talks are not for heavy issues, but rather to connect emotionally with your lifemate at the day's end. Once both partners have completed the statements, discuss what you shared.

When Nothing   34
Really Is Wrong

Check the statements that apply to you: (1) You're very health conscious. (2) If you were to get an unusual pain in your chest, you'd wonder if it were a heart attack. (3) You've done "research" to try to get more information on an illness you had. (4) You read health literature regularly.

If you checked all four statements as applying to you, there's a high likelihood that you are—brace yourself—perfectly normal.

There's a big difference between a person taking an active interest in his health and being a hypochondriac. The latter has real symptoms all right, maybe even real illnesses (usually minor), so he's not a faker. But a hypochondriac blows the significance of his symptoms way out of proportion. It's not just a little ache—every little symptom is something terrifying, a tumor for sure or something just as awful.

The hypochondriac behaves this way because of a psychological problem—called hypochondriasis in the *Diagnostic and Statistical Manual of Mental Disorders* (which is the standard psychiatric reference book). But in some cases it's a condition that can be cured.

An Overused Term

A lot of mentally healthy people, though, are called hypochondriacs for a lot of silly reasons. (Often the accuser is a spouse: "Will you stop acting like a hypochondriac; there's nothing wrong with you!") So with the help of some experts on the subject, let's once and for all establish what kind of behavior does not make you a hypochondriac.

Paying Attention to Vague Symptoms ▶ The human body is subject to all sorts of aches, twitches, creaks, and things that go bump in the night. Hypochondria expert Robert Kellner, M.D., professor of psychiatry at the University of New Mexico, Albuquerque, estimates that in any given week, up to 80 percent of us experience minor physical complaints that have no connection with any disease or disorder. The vast majority of these symptoms are harmless. Most of us ignore them. But if a symptom is out of the ordinary—that is, it persists, it's not like other symptoms you've had, or it's severe—then your concern is perfectly normal and it's a good idea to consult a doctor. It's even a good idea to consult your doctor if you're not sure if a symptom is unusual in the first place. Your physician can help you determine what's wrong, if anything, and how urgent the problem may be.

Developing Symptoms after Reading about a Disease ▶ Reading about the symptoms of hypochondria may make you think you're a hypochondriac. But the odds are that you're not. Reading about an illness or seeing a medical report on TV, then "feeling" some of the symptoms is common among medical students. Many experience sympathy pains resembling symptoms of the disease they're studying at the moment. The symptoms may be triggered by psychological stress. But whereas a hypochondriac fixates on symptoms and remains worried about serious illness, an ordinary person quickly gets over these symptoms.

Asking the Doctor Lots of Questions ▶ There was a time when patients felt they were supposed to be silent and obedient, and any patient who asked plenty of questions was in danger of being labeled a hypochondriac. But that era of the "anything you say, Doc" patient is gone. Nowadays, good doctors understand the importance of patients asking questions about the nature of their illness, about treatment options and risks, about what's going to happen next and why. Getting the answers helps reduce your stress and lets you take a more active role in your own treatment.

Getting a Second Opinion ▶ It's your right to seek another medical opinion (and it's actually encouraged when the first physician recommends surgery or diagnoses a cancer). Sometimes even getting a third or fourth opinion (or more) is reasonable if unanswered questions remain or the diagnosis is an especially tough one.

Whether or not the first doctor says nothing is wrong, make sure the second doctor knows about the first opinion and has access to any tests or pertinent medical records. Many times a family doctor who can't identify the problem will send you to an appropriate specialist.

Switching Doctors ▶ It's perfectly all right to stop going to a doctor you don't like because of conflicts of personality or treatment style. If you feel your doctor doesn't pay enough attention to you during office visits, talk to him or her about it. If the situation doesn't change, you're not being a hypochondriac if you switch to a more user-friendly physician.

Doing Things That Promote Your Own Health ▶ Taking care of yourself and being concerned about your health is most definitely not a marker of hypochondria, no matter what your couch potato friends say. Hypochondriacs are always focusing on disease; people who take care of themselves are focusing on their health. That's the real difference between the two.

Having a Psychosomatic Illness ▶ A psychosomatic malady is a true physical ailment (sometimes debilitating) that's triggered by psychological or emotional problems in some people. The physical symptoms can be verified by a doctor and are as real as can be to the patient—they're not "all in the mind," or imaginary. Peptic ulcer, bronchial asthma, and ulcerative colitis can all be, in some cases, psychosomatic, which is not the same thing as hypochondriacal.

The Real McCoy

"Hypochondria can be viewed as one of two extremes," says Arthur J. Barsky, M.D., associate professor of psychiatry at Harvard Medical School. "At one end there's the stoic, who denies disease and pain. At the other end is the hypochondriac, who exaggerates them. And there are a number of degrees in between." The true hypochondriac has these three characteristics.

■ Morbid fear of disease. None of us wants to get sick, but hypochondriacs live in terror of illness. They respond with immediate alarm to the slightest hint of disease.

■ Preoccupation with bodily symptoms and functions. Hypochondriacs don't just react to unusual sensations— they're obsessed with them and constantly monitor themselves for anything out of the ordinary. They do this without any objective reason for believing that something might be wrong. (Unlike, say, diabetics or people with high blood pressure who have good reason for monitoring blood sugar or blood pressure.)

■ Firm conviction of having a disease. Despite medical reassurance and test results to the contrary, a hypochondriac remains convinced that he or she has a serious disease that remains undetected. In his or her mind, real symptoms (no matter how minor) are sure signs of some terrible disorder.

So hypochondriacs aren't satisfied with a 2nd or 3rd opinion—or a 23rd opinion. And they might not tell the 2nd-through-23rd physicians that they've already been to other doctors. Which means they get the same battery of tests over and over.

That's where the hypochondriac can do a big disservice to himself or herself and others. Normally, when a patient is referred for a second opinion, the physician has access to the test results and diagnosis from the first physician. After examining the patient, the second doctor may have some tests redone to confirm results or may order new tests to look for a different problem. But a second opinion isn't a second opinion if the physician doesn't know there was a first opinion. The doctor wastes his time and the patient's.

Beating Fear of Illness

Knowing something about the cause of hypochondria has helped experts treat it successfully. Hypochondria seems to be fine-tuned early in life. Many hypochondriacs had parents who would become extremely concerned at the first hint of illness. Grown-up hypochondriacs tend to have a low tolerance for pain. And hypochondriacal behavior can sometimes be a symptom of clinical depression and certain panic disorders. In these cases, treating the primary mental disorder causes the hypochondriasis to disappear.

Treating "primary" hypochondriasis is tougher, but clinical results prove it can be done. Generally, treatment consists of evaluating the symptoms (not always easy, since the patients tend to switch doctors frequently) and the physician's continued reassurance when nothing physical is wrong. Many such patients gradually do realize that nothing serious is wrong despite their symptoms because they see that the "condition" they think they have doesn't get worse over time and they don't die.

When a physician's reassurance is not enough, psychiatric help may be necessary. Some patients have changed their beliefs after five to ten sessions with a psychiatrist.

"Hypochondriacs can be helped. Several of the published studies report a positive outcome in a large proportion of patients," says Dr. Kellner. And all the other people who really care about their health can stop wondering whether they're hypochondriacs.

35　Returning from the Depths of Depression

Everyone gets "the blues" when disappointed. And everyone gets depressed over job lay-offs, divorce, the death of a loved one, or other major losses. Sadness is a normal part of life. But when sadness never returns to gladness, it becomes what many authorities call the nation's leading mental health problem, clinical depression.

What Is Depression?

The American Psychiatric Association recognizes several types of clinical depression including major depression, dysthymia (*dis-THIME-ee-ah*), and seasonal affective disorder.

Major Depression ▶ This type typically strikes without any triggering loss, says Michael Freeman, M.D., an assistant clinical professor of psychiatry at the University of California's San Francisco Medical Center. If a trigger can be identified, the sadness is unjustifiably deep. Major depression is a recurring illness that causes gloom so profound the person might not get out of bed, or get dressed, or eat for days at a time. Major depression typically involves several of the following:

■ Apathy and lethargy.

■ Loss of interest in formerly pleasurable activities.

■ Decreased sex drive.

■ A change in appetite, or significant weight loss or gain.

■ Insomnia or significant increase in sleep.

■ Feelings of worthlessness, hopelessness, and/or terrible guilt.

- Difficulty concentrating, or unusual indecisiveness.
- Suicidal thoughts. (See the section, "Danger Signs of Suicide" on page 304.)

Dysthymia ▶ This is similar to major depression, but the symptoms are milder. "Dysthymia is a low-grade, chronic, unremitting depression," Dr. Freeman says. "People with dysthymia can still function, but they're sad sacks."

Seasonal Affective Disorder (SAD) ▶ SAD is often called "winter blues." A reaction to lack of sunlight in winter, it develops in late fall and clears up in early spring. As distance from the equator increases, this condition becomes more common. In the northern hemisphere, December, January, and February are the worst months.

Another illness related to depression is manic-depression or bipolar disorder, which involves major depressive episodes alternating with high-energy periods of wildly unrealistic activity, for example, calling at 3:00 A.M. to demand that you fly to Paris immediately to help stop nuclear terrorists. A major depression often proceeds the first manic episode, Dr. Freeman says.

A Remarkably Common Condition

Depression is so common, it's often called "the common cold of mental health problems." About 5 percent of Americans—some 12 million people—suffer depression.

Authorities estimate that depression costs the nation $20 billion a year for medications, professional care, and lost school and workdays. The toll in human misery is incalculable. The dark cloud of depression has an even darker lining—thoughts of suicide. Each year, tens of thousands of depressed people attempt suicide. An estimated 16,000 succeed. Suicide is now a leading cause of death among teens and young adults.

The Biochemistry of Losses

Clinical depression has recently discovered biochemical roots. Severely depressed people have unusual levels of one hormone (cortisol) and several brain chemicals (serotonin, dopamine, and norepinephrine). These traits may be inherited. In addition, depression tends to run in families, prompting researchers to suspect a genetic connection. But to date, no "depression gene" has been discovered. Authorities also believe that depression runs in families because children pick up depressed parents' gloomy worldview.

Without a family history, deep emotional losses apparently trigger the biochemical changes that cause depression. Profound trauma in early childhood—bitter divorce, the death of a parent, or other deeply disturbing experiences—can set the emotional stage for depression later in life.

Who's at risk? And why?

Relatives ▶ It may be genetics or family socialization, but close relatives of those diagnosed with depression are twice as likely to become seriously depressed as those with no depressed relatives.

Women ▶ Women suffer depression twice as frequently as men. The latest research suggests that severe childhood emotional trauma is one reason. The American Psychological Association's recent Task Force on Women and Depression discovered that 37 percent of depressed women had suffered significant physical or sexual abuse by age 21.

Another reason, the task force suggested, is that women are more likely than men to be socialized into passive, "victim" roles, which leave them feeling powerless and prone to depression. In addition, women must cope with the mood-altering hormonal effects of the menstrual cycle, pregnancy, childbirth, infertility, and/or oral contraceptives.

"Women are also more likely than men to define themselves in terms of their relationships with others," says Eda Spielman, Psy.D., a Boston area clinical psychologist. "As a result, women tend to experience losses more deeply, which makes them more vulnerable to depression."

The Baby Boom Generation ▶ The elderly used to be the group most prone to depression, but no longer. Recent studies suggest that the post–World War II generation is currently at greatest risk. Researchers theorize that depression in many baby boomers may be a reaction to the emotional disruptions of growing up in 1950s' and 1960s' America—unprecedented rates of divorce and relocation, leading to losses of family, friends, and community.

In addition, the baby boom generation came of age during a time of record economic expansion, which created great expectations of wealth and success, according to Gerald Klerman, M.D., a professor of psychiatry at Cornell University Medical College in New York. But their enormous numbers also meant unprecedented competition for schools, jobs, and housing. And the nation's economic problems have left many of their dreams unfulfilled. "Risk of depression increases," Dr. Klerman says, "when people feel a gap between what they expect and what they get. Unfulfilled expectations cause disappointment, frustration, loss of self-esteem . . . and sometimes depression."

But those who have achieved success are by no means immune to depression. In today's corporate pressure cooker, the emotional price of success can also be quite high.

Children ▶ Depression is not common in young children, but abuse, losses, and having a seriously depressed parent increase the risk.

"Depressed children may not show obvious sadness," Dr. Spielman says. "Their symptoms tend to be behav-

301
■

ioral." Look for unusual irritability, aggressive outbursts, and problems at school.

Teens ▶ In recent years, depression has become more common among teens. "Adolescence is a difficult period," Dr. Spielman explains. "Teens experience major hormonal changes. They have higher highs and lower lows. And they're loosening family ties, but not yet established as individuals." This combination can lead to deeply emotional reactions to major losses.

To identify depression in teens, look for problems at school, inability to bounce back after disappointments, or any sudden change in mood or behavior that doesn't make sense. Be extra-vigilant if anyone the adolescent knows attempts or commits suicide.

The Elderly ▶ Depression in older people is often a reaction to physical deterioration and the loss of friends, family, and rewarding activities. "Being lonely, isolated, and infirm can be very depressing," Dr. Freeman says.

Unexplained crying is often a clue. Also, look for a combination of vague physical symptoms, for example, headache, difficulty swallowing, chest pain, and upset stomach. Once other illnesses have been ruled out, depression is a real possibility.

City Residents ▶ For reasons that remain unclear, major depression is more common in urban than rural areas, but other forms of depression don't exhibit this pattern.

Rediscovering the Joy in Life

Tragically, only about one-third of those suffering what author and depression survivor William Styron recently called "the howling tempest in the brain" ever seek treatment. The myth is that people who can't climb out of the emotional quicksand lack strength of character.

But "depression is not a moral weakness," Dr. Freeman says. "It's a medical condition with clear biological roots."

It's also increasingly treatable—a major psychiatric triumph. About 80 percent of depression sufferers can now be treated successfully, typically with a combination of the following therapies.

Cognitive Restructuring ▶ You can't talk yourself out of depression, but you can stop talking yourself deeper into it. Cognitive therapy empowers people to recognize—and correct—depressive thinking. If you make a mistake at work, you might think: "I'm hopelessly incompetent," and slide toward depression. That's "awfulizing," a thought distortion that magnifies minor upsets into catastrophes. With cognitive therapy, the reaction changes: "Okay, I made a mistake. Everyone makes mistakes. Fortunately, my boss and co-workers know I don't make many. And I can fix this one easily." A National Institute of Mental Health (NIMH) study showed that after 16 weeks of cognitive restructuring training, 51 percent of those with mild to moderate depression reported significant improvement. "Cognitive therapy also lends itself to self-help," Dr. Freeman says.

Psychotherapy ▶ Long-term Freudian psychoanalysis has been largely replaced by shorter-term "talk therapies." The NIMH study showed that after 16 weeks of psychotherapy, 55 percent of those with mild to moderate depression reported significant improvement. How long is long enough? "For most major depressive episodes," Dr. Freeman says, "four to five months is usually about right."

Medications ▶ These include tricyclic antidepressants (Elavil, Tofranil, etc.), monoamine oxidase (MAO) inhibitors (Marplan, Nardil, etc.), and the newest drug, fluoxetine (Prozac). Studies show they help about 80 percent of those with moderate to severe depression. All antidepressant medications may cause side effects—some

303
■

possibly severe—so dosages must be monitored closely by a physician, ideally by a psychiatrist experienced in their use. Drug treatment typically lasts four to eight months.

Phototherapy ▶ Those with SAD sit in front of bright fluorescent lights for several hours a day. Studies show that light therapy lifts the spirits of 60 to 80 percent of those with winter depression. Midwinter tropical vacations also help. After you return, the emotional benefits typically last a week or two.

In addition, Dr. Freeman advocates other depression relievers: exercise, spending time in the sun, and making time for life's little pleasures. "Try to do something fun every day," he advises.

Educate the Whole Family

The misery of depression extends beyond those suffering it to their families and friends. Depressed people often frustrate and alienate those around them. "Try not to take it personally," Dr. Freeman says. He advises those involved with depressed people to learn more about the condition, and encourage the sufferer to get treated as quickly as possible.

Dr. Spielman urges friends and relatives to guard against falling victim to depression themselves: "Stay involved with other people. Don't become isolated." She also advises reassuring the children of depressed parents that the illness is not their fault. "Otherwise," she says, "children may blame themselves for the parent's condition, feel guilty, and become more vulnerable to depression."

Danger Signs of Suicide

Depression often leads to suicide attempts. You don't have to be a physician or psychologist to recognize the danger signs of suicide, Dr. Freeman says. If anyone you

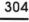

know starts saying or doing any of the following, urge the person to seek help. Or call your physician or a local mental health agency.

Words ▶ "Life isn't worth living." "Maybe things would be better if I weren't around." "Sometimes I just want to go to sleep and not wake up." "Who do you think would come to my funeral?" "I'm thinking about killing myself."

Actions ▶ Unusual apathy, lethargy, hopelessness, withdrawal, or loss of appetite; saying goodbye in a way that implies the person won't see you again; giving away valued personal property; any significant self-injury; taking drug overdoses "accidentally."

Index